Intermittent Fasting for Women

"The Definite Guide to Lose Your Weight and Burn Fat, the Easiest Way to Improve Your Life"

Mary Di Marzio

Table of Contents

Intermittent Fasting for Women

permission from the publisher. All rights reserved.

themselves, not affiliated with this document.

CHAPTER ONE

INTERMITTENT FASTING

Intermittent fasting (IF) refers to a nutritional pattern that involves eating for a long time or severely limiting calories. There are many different subgroups with intermittent fasting and each variation in the duration of fasting; some for hours, others for days. This has become a trending topic in the scientific community because of all the potential benefits of fitness and health discovered.

➢ **What is Intermittent Fasting (IF)?**
Fasting or voluntary withdrawal of food has been practiced worldwide for centuries. From time to time, fasting to improve health is relatively new. Intermediate publication involves limiting food consumption for a given period and does not include any changes in the food you eat. Currently, the

most common protocols for IF are to fast daily, 16 hours a day, all day, one or two days a week. From time to time, fasting can be considered as a natural diet to which humans were conceived, and it goes back to our ancestors of Palaeolithic hunters and gatherers. An existing model of a planned intermittent fasting program could help improve many aspects of health, from body composition to longevity and aging. Although contrary to the norms of our culture and our typical daily routine, science may indicate that the frequency of meals and a longer duration of fasting are the optimal alternative to the healthy model of breakfast, lunch, and dinner. Here are two common myths related to occasional fasting.

Myth 1: "Eat three meals a day", this rule, common in Western society, was not developed based on evidence of better health, but was accepted as a typical model for immigrants and has finally become standard. Not only are models of three meals a day lacking scientific reasoning, but recent studies may also show that fewer meals and more fasting are optimal for human health.

One study found that one meal a day with the same amount of calories was better for weight loss and body composition than three meals a day. This discovery is a central term extrapolated to the fasting publication, and those who opt for the IF may find it better to eat one to two meals a day.

Myth 2: "I need breakfast", the most important meal of the day. Many false claims have been made about the absolute need for daily breakfast. The most common charges are "breakfast increases metabolism" and "breakfast decreases food intake later in the day". These statements were rejected and studied for 16 weeks, and the results showed that skipping breakfast does not reduce metabolism and does not increase food intake at lunch and dinner. It is still possible to make protocols with occasional fasts while resuming breakfast. Anyways, some people find it easier to take late breakfast or ignore it completely, and this common myth should not be distracted.

➢ **Types of Intermitting Fasting (IF):**
The broken publication comes in different forms, and each of them may have a specific

set of unique advantages. Every kind of intermittent fasting has variations in the proportion of fasting and diet. The benefits and effectiveness of these different protocols can vary individually, and it is crucial to determine which one is best for you. The most common types of IF are alternative daily fasting, limited time feeding, and modified fasting.

➢ Fasting Alternate Day:

This approach alternately involves days without calories (food or drinks), with days free of meals or with meals. This plan has been shown to help you lose weight, improve blood cholesterol and triglyceride levels, and improve markers of inflammation in your blood.

The main disadvantage of this form of intermittent fasting is that it is more difficult to bear because of the hunger reported during the fasting days.

➢ Modified Fasting:

Modified fasting is a protocol with planned fasting days, but fasting days allow for some consumption of food. In general, 20 to 25%

of ordinary calories can be consumed on fasting days. Therefore, if you regularly consume 2,000 calories a day, you will be allowed to consume between 400 to 500 calories on fasting days. Part of this 5:2 diet is the number of days without fasting and fasting. So, in this diet, I would typically eat for five consecutive days, then fast or limit my calories to 20-25% for two days straight.

This protocol is ideal for weight loss, body composition and can also help regulate blood sugar, lipids and inflammation. Studies have shown that the 5:2 contract is beneficial for weight loss, to improve/reduce markers of inflammation in the blood and to show signs of improvement in insulin resistance. In animal studies, this modified fasting diet of 5:2 resulted in decreased fat, decreased hunger hormone (leptin) and increased protein levels to improve body fat. Fat burning and regulation of blood sugar (adiponectin).

The modified 5:2 fasting protocol is usual to follow and has some harmful side effects, including hunger, loss of energy, and some irritability at the beginning of the program.

Intermittent Fasting for Women

In contrast, studies have also noted improvements such as decreased tension, decreased anger, reduced fatigue, improved self-confidence, and improved mood.

➢ Time-Restricted Feeding:

If you know someone who told you to fast intermittently, it is likely to take the form of a diet that is limited in time. It is a type of occasional fast that is used daily and involves consuming calories for only a small portion of the day and fasting for the rest. Daily fasting intervals in the restricted diet range from 12 to 20 hours, with the most common method being 16/8 i.e., fasting 16 hours, calorie intake 8 hours). For this protocol, the time of day does not matter as long as you starve consecutively and only eat during the period allowed. For example, in a feeding program limited to 16/8, a person can bite their first meal at 7 o'clock. And the last meal at 3 pm (fast between 3 pm and 7 pm), while the other person can have their first meal at 1 pm. and the last meal at 9 pm. (fast from 13h to 21h). This protocol should be implemented daily for long periods and is very flexible as long as it remains in the quick/meal.

Food with a time limit is one of the most natural methods to follow from time to time. Its use, combined with a daily schedule of work and sleep, can help you achieve optimal metabolic function. Diet over time is limited by an excellent program of weight loss and weight gain, as well as by some other health benefits. Several human experiences have shown significant weight loss, decreased blood glucose in the evening, and improved cholesterol without altering perceived tension, depression, anger, fatigue, or confusion. Some other preliminary results from animal studies have shown a limited temporal regimen protecting against obesity, high insulin stage, fatty liver disease, and inflammation.

Simple administration and promising results of a time-limited diet could make it an excellent option for weight loss and chronic disease prevention/management. When implementing this protocol, it may be wise to start with a small portion of your diet, such as 12/12 hours and possibly work up to 16/8 hours.

> **Questions Common About Intermitting Fasting:**

Are there foods or drinks that I can consume during intermittent fasting? If you are not on a modified fasting diet 5:2 (mentioned above), you should not eat or drink anything that contains calories. Water, black coffee and any non-calorie food/drink can be eaten during fasting. Adequate water intake is crucial during the IF, and some experts suggest that consuming black coffee during fasting helps reduce hunger.

> **If You Want the Benefits:**

Research on intermittent fasting is in its infancy, but the potential for weight loss and treatment of some chronic diseases remains considerable.

To conclude, here are some possible advantages of the occasional edition:

Presented in Human Sciences:

1. Weight loss.

2. Improves blood lipid markers such as cholesterol.

3. Reduce inflammation.

4. Reduce stress and improve self-confidence.

5. Better mood.

Presented in Animal Studies:

1. Reduces body fat.

2. Reduces hormone levels soften leptin.

3. Improves insulin levels.

4. Protects against obesity, fatty liver disease and inflammation.

5. Longevity.

➤ Fasting and Female Hormone:

In the grand scheme of the health decisions of your life, experimenting with the IF seems minimal, isn't it? Unfortunately, for some women; at least, it appears that small choices can have significant effects.

It turns out that hormones that regulate essential functions such as ovulation are susceptible to energy intake.

In both men and women, the cooperative functioning of the hypothalamicpituitarygonadal (HPG) axis of the three endocrine glands plays the role of controller of air traffic.

First, the hypothalamus releases gonadotropin releasing hormone (GnRH).

This tells the pituitary gland to release luteinizing hormone (LH) and follicle-stimulating hormone (FSH).

LH and FSH act on the gonadal (also called testes or ovaries).

In women, this triggers the output of estrogen and progesterone, necessary for the release of the mature egg (ovulation) and support for pregnancy.

In men, this triggers testosterone production and sperm production.

Because this chain of reactions occurs in a specific and regular cycle in women, GnRH impulses must be timed accurately, that is, everything can become uncontrollable.

GnRH pulses appear to be very sensitive to environmental factors and can be expelled on an empty stomach.

Even short-term hunger (for example, three days) changes hormonal impulses in some women.

It is even proven that the absence of a regular meal, (although it is not a necessity in itself), can alert our antennas so that our body becomes ready to react quickly to changes in energy supply if it continues.

This may be why some women get along well with the SI, while others have problems.

> **Why does IF affect Female Hormones more than Male Hormones?**

We are not sure on this. Nevertheless, it could have something to do with Kisspeptin, a protein-like molecule that neurons use to communicate with each other (and do essential things).

Kisspeptin promotes the production of GnRH in both sexes, and we know that it is sensitive to leptin, insulin, and ghrelin, hormones that regulate and respond to hunger and satiety.

Interestingly, mammalian females have more kisspeptin than men. A more significant number of kisspeptin neurons may indicate a higher sensitivity to changes in the energy balance.

This could be one of the signs why the physical production of kisspeptin in women decreases more rapidly, which is why, their GnRH does not work.

The Methods:

The subjects included ten male rats and ten normal female rats.

Half of the rats ate when they wanted.

The other half of the meal was served only every other day. In between meals, they took food and fasted.

It lasted 12 weeks, the equivalent of ten years of human life.

The Results:

At the end of 12 weeks, female rats with voices lost 19% of their weight, blood sugar was lower, and their ovaries decreased.

In general, the experiment affected the hormones of female rats more significantly than males.

While kisspeptin production was reduced in female rats, LH collapsed in females, while estradiol, a hormone that inhibits GnRH in humans, increased fourfold.

The leptin hormone of appetite was six times lower than that of a woman who usually feeds.

The experiment only took 10 to 15 days to break the reproductive cycle.

In other words, the female rat hormones, as well as the reproduction and regulation of appetite, were entirely out of control.

What does this mean for people?

It's hard to say. But according to what we know about the HPG axis, kisspeptin, the link between hormones and appetite and women's sensitivity to environmental factors, it is possible that fasting can have an equally dramatic effect on women as well.

Fertility; compatible with metabolism.

You may be thinking: what is the problem if kisspeptin falls and you miss specific rules? Anyways, you do not have any children soon.

Here is the Thing.

The female reproductive system and metabolism are intensely linked. If you miss your period, you can bet that many hormones are changed, not just those that help you get pregnant.

Take this picture.

Women generally, eat less protein than men. Fasting women consume even less.

Consuming less protein means eating fewer amino acids.

Amino acids are essential for estrogen receptor activation and the synthesis of insulin-like growth factor (IGF-1) in the liver. IGF-1 causes a thickening of the lining of the uterine wall and advances the reproductive cycle.

A low protein diet can, therefore, reduce fertility. (Not to mention the sexy weather).

And most importantly, estrogen is not just for reproduction.

We have estrogen receptors throughout the body, including the brain, gastrointestinal tract and bones. Change your balance in estrogen and change your metabolic function everywhere; cognition, mood, digestion, recovery, protein recovery, bone formation.

In terms of appetite and energy balance, estrogen works in several ways.

First, in your brain, estrogen changes the peptides that tell you to feel full (cholecystokinin) or hungry (ghrelin).

In the hypothalamus, estrogen also stimulates neurons that stop the production of appetite-regulating peptides.

Do something that lowers your estrogen levels, and you may be much hungrier and eat much more than during under normal circumstances.

Estrogens are therefore essential regulators of metabolism.

Yes, the estrogen; plural. Because the proportions of estrogen metabolites (estriol, estradiol and estrone) change over time, before menopause, estradiol is an excellent player. After menopause, the estrone remains pretty much the same thing.

The exact functions of each of these estrogens remain unclear. But some theorise that a decrease in estradiol can trigger a multiple in fat storage. Why since fat is used to make estradiol?

The men walk, looking tired, and you fight with your belly. In the event that you are a woman, you ought not to stress over your stomach in the sink.

A low energy diet can affect fertility in women. Overweight is a reproductive disability. The female body is well suited to any threat of energy and productivity.

When you think about it, it has an evolutionary meaning.

Human females are unique in the world of mammals. Understand this: almost all the other mammals can abort or suspend their pregnancy at any time. You know it from high school health class: women cannot do it.

In humans, the placenta violates the mother's blood vessels, and the fetus has complete control.

Your baby may block the action of insulin to collect more glucose. The fetus can even dilate the mother's blood vessels, adjusting her blood pressure to get more nutrients.

This baby is determined to survive, no matter how much it costs the mother. This phenomenon, which scientists have compared to the virus-host relationship, is known as "Mother-fetus Conflict".

Once pregnant, a woman can no longer tell the fetus to stop growing. The result: fertility at the wrong time, as during a famine, could be fatal.

It is not surprising that the reproductive path is sensitive to multilevel metabolic signals.

How does the body "know"? Okay, a woman's hormonal balance is particularly sensitive to the amount, the frequency, and what we eat. But how do our bodies "know" when they have a little food?

For many years, scientists have thought that a woman's body fat percentage regulates her reproductive system.

The idea was that if their fat intake fell below a certain percentage (we can reasonably assume about 11%), the hormones would decompose and their period would end. Boom! No risk of pregnancy.

It makes a lot of sense. If there is not much to eat, you will lose body fat over time.

But the situation is more complicated than that. Finally, the availability of food can change quickly. As you probably already know, if you have ever tried to lose weight, body fat often takes a long time to fall, even if you eat fewer calories.

Meanwhile, women who are not particularly thin can also stop ovulating and losing their periods.

For this reason, scientists have noticed that the overall energy balance may be more critical in the process than the percentage of body fat per person.

Of course, occasional fasting can be generalized. And maybe your brother, boyfriend, husband or even your father is considered an essential asset for fitness and health.

But women are different from men, and our bodies have different needs.

Listen to your body. And do what suit you the best.

Stressors and Energy Balance.

In particular, the negative hormonal balance in women may be due to the hormonal domino effect we have discussed. And it's not just the amount of food you eat.

The negative energy balance can be the result of:

- too small food.
- poor nutrition.
- too much exercise.
- too much stress.
- disease, infection, chronic inflammation.
- very little rest and recovery.

We can even use energy reserves trying to keep us warm.

Any combination of these stresses could be okay to put her in a negative energy balance and stop ovulation: training for a marathon, taking care of the flu, too many consecutive days at the gym without enough fruits and vegetables, to fast from time to time and kick my ass to pay the mortgage.

Thinking, have you had a relationship with the payment of your mortgage? Bet psychological stress can play a role in disrupting our hormonal balance. Our bodies cannot distinguish a real threat from something imaginary generated by our thoughts and feelings. (How to worry about getting abs). The stress hormone, cortisol, inhibits our friend's GnRH and inhibits the production of estrogen and progesterone in the ovaries.

Meanwhile, progesterone becomes cortisol during stress, so more cortisol means less progesterone. This directs to estrogen dominance in the HPG axis. This could be around 30% fat. But if your energy balance remains long enough negative, especially if you are stressed, reproduction stops.

What to do now? As we know, intermittent fasting is likely to affect reproductive health if it is perceived as a significant stressor by the body. Everything that affects your reproductive health affects your health and your overall fitness. Even if you do not mean to have children.

But intermittent fasting protocols vary, and some are much more extreme than others. And elements such as your age, your nutritional status, the time you spend in your life, and other stresses in your life, including training, are also likely relevant.

> **Advice on Intermittent Fasting?**

Given the little that remains to be clarified, I would suggest a conservative approach.

If you want to test the IF, start with a flexible protocol and be attentive to the evolution of the situation.

When you Stop Intermittent Fasting (IF):

- your menstrual cycle stops or becomes irregular.
- have trouble falling asleep.
- your hair falls.
- you start to develop dry skin or acne.
- you realise that you cannot recover so quickly after training.
- wounds need healing time or you can have all insects expelled.
- reduce stress tolerance.
- moods begin to change.
- your heart starts to beat in a strange way.
- interest in romance fails (and their female roles stop enjoying it when it happens).
- your digestion slows down considerably.
- you always seem to be cold.

Fasting is not for everyone. The truth is that some women should not even bother to experiment. Do not try IF if:

- you are pregnant.
- You have a history of eating disorders.
- you are chronically stressed.
- you do not sleep well.
- you are new to diet and exercise.

Pregnant women have higher energy needs. So, if you start a family, fasting is not a good idea.

Same thing if you are under chronic stress or if you are not sleeping well. Your body needs care, not extra weight.

And if you've ever had problems with your eating disorder, you probably know that the fasting protocol can lead you on a path that could cause you more problems. Why play with your health? There are other ways to obtain look benefits. If you are new to diet and exercise, this may seem like a quick fix to weight loss. But it would be much wiser to get rid of any nutritional deficiency before you begin to experience fasting. Start with a healthy diet base first.

What if the job is not for you?

How can you integrate and lose weight if fasting occasionally is not a good option for you? It's simple. Learn the basics of proper nutrition. This is by far the right thing to do for your health and fitness.

Cook and eat whole foods, exercise regularly, be consistent and if you need help with all this, hire a coach.

➢ **Tips for Intermittent Fasting:**
It can be challenging to follow an informal program of publications.

- The following tips can help people stay on track and maximise the benefits of intermittent fasting. Avoid the obsession with food. Plan for many distractions during the fasting days to avoid thinking of food, such as going to the cinema or reading newspaper.
- Rest and Relax. Avoid strenuous activities on days of fasting, although

light exercises such as yoga can be helpful. Create any amount of calories if your chosen plan allows you to consume a few calories during the fasting period, choose foods that are rich in nutrients, rich in protein, fibre and healthy fats. E.g. beans, lentils, eggs, fish, nuts and avocados.

- Eat large amounts of food. Choose an abundant but low-calorie diet that includes popcorn, raw vegetables, and fruits that are too rich in water, such as grapes and melons.
- Increased taste without calories. Season with garlic, herbs, spices or vinegar. These foods lack calories, but they are full of flavour, which can help reduce hunger.
- Choose nutrient-rich foods after fasting. Eating foods high in fibre, vitamins, minerals and other nutrients helps maintain blood glucose levels and prevent nutritional deficiencies. A balanced diet will also add to weight loss and overall health.

Stay hydrated during the day, drink plenty of water without calories, such as herbal teas.

> Decide First if it's for You.

Although there are some exciting benefits, IF is not for everyone. Your exercise, your nutrition experience and lifestyle should determine whether you are testing the IF. If you are new to yoga and nutrition, I recommend you to first learn the basics.

> **Start Slowly, Small and Gradually.**

If you decide to try the IF, nothing presses. Choose a small thing to work on, even if it's a regular meal adjustment for an hour. Try to see how it goes.

Focus on common IS approaches instead of getting stuck in the details.

Sometimes you eat, sometimes you don't. That adds. Remain flexible, get to know yourself, look at your experiences.

To be a scientist; start, collect data, get information, and draw conclusions that you will use to guide future actions. Do what's right for you.

➢ **Take time.**

You don't need to put yourself in a hurry. Especially since we usually need a few weeks to adapt to our new program. Wait for the ups and downs.

They happen; it's part of life and process. If you stay open and do not panic during an "accident", you will discover how to have more "ups".

Think about what you want from IF. Focus on the calibre of the process, not the outcome.

IF is a great way to:

- deepen the psychological and physical experience of real hunger.
- know the difference between "head hunger" and "body hunger".
- to learn not to fear hunger.
- improve insulin sensitivity and recalibrate the use of fuel stored in your body.
- respect the procedure and the privilege of eating.
- find out more about your own body.

Intermittent Fasting for Women

- lose fat if you are careful.

Take a break from your meal preparation and your commitment to eating.

IF is not healthy if:

- use the excuse of "health" as a mean of causing eating disorders and strictly controlling your food intake (which is the same).
- to fast too often, too long.
- you are doing too much physical activity or not getting enough sleep (that is, you are undergoing too much physiological stress).
- use many supplements, legal or otherwise, to kill your appetite quickly.
- you are obsessed with food and overeat during your fasting periods.
- use IF as a means of "catching up" with poor food choices or excessive consumption of food.

What you eat is as important as what you do not know.

Get nutritional basics first. Eat quality food in the right quantities, at the right time. For most people, this is enough for a good shape. Not, if necessary.

For more information, check out our five-day fat loss course in the resources section.

Respect the signals of your body. Pay attention to what your body tells you.

These include:

- drastic changes in appetite, hunger and satiety, including cravings.
- quality of sleep.
- energy levels and sports performance.
- mood and mental/emotional health.
- immunity.
- blood profile.
- hormonal health.

How you look?

Exercise, but do not overdo it.

We recommend combining exercise and IF to get the most out of it. Just do not do too much.

Think about what's going on in your life.

Think of:

- how much exercise/training do you do and how intensively.
- how do you rest and recover?
- to what extent does this fit into your current and healthy social activities.
- what other demands and stressful life has to offer.

Remember: IF is one of many restoration styles that work. But this "works" only when it is intermittent, flexible, and part of its usual routine, it is not a duty, it is not a constant source of physical and psychological stress.

➢ **Ways to get an Intermittent Fast:** There are different methods of casual fasting, and people prefer different styles. Read on to learn seven different ways to reach occasional publications.

1. Quick 12 hours a day:

The rules of this diet are simple. The person must decide each day and comply with the fasting window for 12 hours.

According to some researchers, fasting for 10 to 16 hours can cause to burn fat stores into energy, releasing ketones into the bloodstream. This should encourage weight loss.

This type of open publishing plan can be a good option for beginners. Indeed, the fasting window being relatively small, many fasts occur during sleep, and a person can consume the same amount of calories each day.

The easiest way to achieve a 12-hour fast is to include a period of sleep in the electric window.

For example, some people may decide to fast between 19:00 and 7 am. They must finish their dinner before 7 PM and wait until 7 AM for breakfast, but most of the time they sleep in between.

2. Post 16 hours:

Fasting 16 hours a day without stopping for 8 hours is called the 16:8 or Leangains diet.

During the 16/8 diet, men fast 16 hours a day and women 14 hours. This type of intermittent speed can be useful to anyone who has already tried the 12-hour rate without seeing the benefit.

With this post, people usually finish their dinner at 8 pm, and then skip breakfast the next day without eating again until noon.

A trusted source study in mice found that limiting their time to 8 hours protected them from obesity, inflammation, diabetes, and liver disease, even when they consumed the same amount of total calories than the mice they ate when they wanted to.

3. Fast two days a week:

People on a 5:2 diet eat standard amounts of healthy foods for five days and the other two days reduce their caloric intake.

During the two days of fasting, men consume 600 calories and women consume 500 calories.

Usually, fasting days are separated from the week. For example, they can fast on Mondays and Thursdays, and they typically eat other days. There must be at least one day without fasting between the days of fasting.

There is little research on the 5:2 diet, also called a fast diet. A trusted source study of 107 overweight or obese women found that a two-weekly calorie restriction and a reduction in calories resulted in a similar weight reduction.

The investigation likewise found that this eating routine diminished insulin levels and improved insulin sensitivity in participants.

A small study analysed the effects of this fasting style on 23 overweight women. During the menstrual cycle, women lost 4.8% of their body weight and 8.0% of their total body fat. However, after five days of healthy eating, these measures have returned to normal for most women.

4. Alternative Daily Publication:

There are several variations of a fasting plan during the second day, which include fasting every other day.

For some people, daily fasting means altogether avoiding solid foods on days of fasting, while others allow up to 500 calories. On meal days, people often choose to eat as much as they want.

One study, Trusted Source, indicates that alternative fasting is effective for weight loss and heart health in healthy and overweight individuals. The researchers found that 32 participants lost an average of 5.2 kg (kg), a little over 11 kilograms in 12 weeks.

Alternative fasting during the day is a relatively extreme form of intermittent fasting and may not be suitable for beginners or people with specific health problems. It can also be challenging to maintain this publication in the long run.

> **Weekly Fast of 24 hours:**

Complete fasting 1 or 2 days a week, known as the "eat, stop eating" diet, means not eating food at the same time for 24 hours. Numerous individuals fast quick from breakfast to breakfast or lunch to lunch. People who follow this diet can drink water, tea and other non-calorie beverages during fasting.

People should return to regular fasting eating habits for days. Eating in this way reduces its overall caloric intake but does not limit the specific foods that are consumed.

Fasting for 24 hours can be challenging and can cause fatigue, headaches or excitability. Many people find that these consequences become less utmost over time, as the body adapts to this new diet.

People can benefit from trying 12 to 16 hours before moving on to 24 hours.

➢ **Skip the Food:**
This flexible approach to casual display may be suitable for beginners. Sometimes it involves skipping meals.

People can choose foods to avoid, based on their hunger or their time limit. However, it is crucial to eat healthy foods at every meal.

Missed meals will likely be more successful when people monitor and respond to hunger signals in their bodies. Generally, people who use this style of casual fasting eat when they are hungry and skip meals when they are not. For some, this may seem more natural than other methods of fasting.

➢ **The Warrior Regime:**
The Warrior Diet is a comparatively extreme form of occasional fasting.

The diet of a warrior is to eat very little, usually a few portions of raw fruits and vegetables, more than 20 hours of fasting, then to take a healthy meal in the evening. The consumption window is usually around 4 hours.

This form of fasting can be better for people who have already tried other types of occasional fasting. Supporters of dietary warriors claim that humans are the natural food of the night and that eating at night allows the body to obtain nutrients that match their circadian rhythms.

During the four-hour feeding phase, people should be sure to consume a lot of vegetables, proteins and healthy fats. They should also include carbohydrates.

Although it is possible to eat certain foods during fasting, it can be challenging to follow strict guidelines regarding the timing and foods to consume for a long time. Also, some people have difficulty eating such a big meal, near to sleep.

There is also a risk that people who follow this diet do not eat enough nutrients, such as fibre. This can increase your risk of cancer and affect your digestive and immune health.

For women who wish to lose weight, occasional fasting may seem like a great option, but many people want to know if women should fast. Is casual fasting effective for women? Several critical studies of intermittent fasting can help us better understand this exciting new food trend.

From time to time, fasting is also a daily alternative, although there are certain variations in this diet. The United States Journal of Clinical Nutrition recently conducted a study of 16 obese men and women in a 10-week program. During the fast, participants consumed up to 25% of their estimated energy needs. The rest of the time, they received nutritional advice but did not receive specific instructions during this time.

As expected, the participants lost weight because of this study, but some specific changes made the researchers enjoyable. All subjects continued to be obese after only ten weeks but showed improvement in cholesterol, LDL cholesterol, triglycerides, and systolic blood pressure. The exciting discovery is that most people must lose more weight than these participants before seeing the same changes. It was a fascinating discovery that prompted a significant number of people to try to fast.

Sometimes fasting in women has beneficial effects. What is especially vital for women trying to lose weight is that they have a much higher proportion of fat in their bodies. In trying to lose weight, the body burns primarily in carbohydrate stores for the first 6 hours and then starts burning fat. Women who need a healthy diet and exercise program may have difficulty with stubborn fat, but fasting is a realistic alternative.

> **Intermittent Fast for Women over Fifty:**

Our body and our metabolism change when we reach menopause. One of the most critical changes that women over fifty have experienced is that they have a slower metabolism and are starting to gain weight. However, fasting can be a great way to reverse and prevent weight gain. Studies have shown that this model of fasting helps regulate appetite and that people who follow it regularly do not feel the same desire as others. If you are over fifty and try to adapt to your slower metabolism, intermittent fasting can help you avoid overeating every day.

At the age of fifty, your body also begins to develop certain chronic conditions such as high cholesterol and high blood pressure. It has been shown that occasional fasting lowers both cholesterol and blood pressure, even without losing a lot of weight. If you notice that your number is increasing every year at the doctor's, you may be able to reduce it again, on an empty stomach, even without losing a lot of weight.

Sometimes fasting may not be a good idea for all women. Anyone with a specific medical condition or who is prone to hypoglycaemia should consult a doctor. However, this new nutritional trend has particular benefits for women who naturally store more fat in the body and may have trouble getting rid of these fat stores.

This is something you can use to improve your overall quality of life in many ways. And as a result, we help you bring more to the community you belong to.

Intermittent Fasting:

You may have heard of an occasional publication. It is a relatively simple nutritional intervention that is widely used, and it can add it with great success. This includes dividing your 24 hours a day into two states or basic categories.

"Fast" or "Fast" status: (between 18 and 48 hours)

"Feed" or "Feed" status:

First, let's look at the status of your message. The time varies from 16:00 to 48:00. Recently, I played with a 16-hour booth, and I also had some experiences with a 24-hour clock.

To begin, you will usually have dinner at 19h or 20h. He would then enrol in his fast for the next 16 to 18 hours for this example. So you get up the next day, and you eventually have morning training or preparation for work.

Side note: if you work in the morning, I will not do it on exercise days, but once a week. I prefer this cardio day only or once a week of resistance training.

Then you will see you eat your first meal at around 11 o'clock at 1 pm that day.

What to consider when publishing:

- Irritability possible.
- Greater need for water consumption.
- The most outstanding ability to distinguish false hunger from real hunger.

- High caloric deficit and restoration of hormonal fat burning by the body.
- The need to consume amino acids during the "fasting state" (especially before and after the morning "fasting" exercises).
- Increased need for a delicious and balanced meal when you are not hungry.

Now let's see the power state.

This period will only last 6 to 10 hours, depending on your last meal of the day. During this time, it is advisable to consume your three main meals. You still have your breakfast, also known as (Break the Fast), only after your routine. You cannot include your typical breakfast meal, but you can do it if it's your choice. Each meal will be of adequate size and will allow you to strengthen the next day.

What to consider when eating or eating:

If you are exercising in the afternoon, try to keep your carbohydrates moderate to low for pre-workout meals. After this night exercise, take large carbohydrate meals to end the day and return to a nutritious state.

Do not be fooled by junk food for the first meal after fasting, which will erase all the sound coming from fasting.

Meals should be the right size and serving size. Listen to your body and always wait 15 to 20 minutes after the meal to see if you need more food. This is what usually takes a meal to reach the stomach and its sensory receptors that indicate hunger.

Advantages and disadvantages of intermittent fasting + general guidelines:

- Pro: creates a significant calorie deficit.
- Pro: Increases fat and calories burned.
- Pro: Increases your ability to identify true and false feelings of hunger.
- Pro: You do not have to eat every 2-3 hours, which can be painful.
- Pro: Increased energy levels and metabolism.
- Cons: Women have problems with this diet.

- Cons: It takes less time to get used to it.
- Cons: You sometimes feel flat, but it is not often reported.

CHAPTER TWO

INTERMITTENT FASTING WEIGHT LOSS

> What Distinguishes an Intermitting Fasting Assignment?

Intermittent weight loss testing is one of the most effective ways to lose weight. Ideas about accidental weight loss become a challenge for most beliefs about weight loss. Those asking for new ways to lose weight quickly adopted their views.

> **What is Intermitting Fasting Weight Loss?**

Let me begin by saying that the intermitting fast is not a diet. You are probably tired of trying anything with the word "diet" when it comes to losing weight. From time to time, fasting is a diet that involves a structured program where you eat, and when you do not eat. You can structure your application as you like if you can manage it quickly throughout the day. I recommend fasting 12 full hours before eating. You can then continue the publication period while keeping the program.

➤ What Makes It Different?

If you have tried to lose weight, you have probably tried a diet like the Atkins diet based on the theory of frequent eating. Supporters of these diets told him to eat frequently throughout the day. The idea was that the more you eat, the faster your metabolism will be. The quicker your metabolism, the fatter you lose. Of course, you know that the more you eat, the more you want to eat, and the more your weight is maintained. When you are in a casual program, you will need to reduce the frequency of your meals. Sometimes you have to do it without breakfast.

➤ Ask More:

You probably sleep for about 6 to 8 hours. Meanwhile, your body is fasting. When your body is fasting, it usually produces more insulin. More insulin in your body makes your body more sensitive to insulin. When you increase the insulin sensitivity in your body, you lose more fat. The great benefit of the intermittent weight loss test is that you skip breakfast to prolong the period of insulin sensitivity of your body. This means that your body will be in fat loss mode for a prolonged period. You will lose more pounds.

Prolonged fasting also has a positive effect on growth hormone levels in your body. When you skip breakfast or eat for a while, your body produces growth hormone. Growth hormone is what you want your body to create when you are trying to lose weight. It's merely because growth hormone promotes weight loss in your body. When working on an occasional weight loss program, your growth hormone level is usually at its peak. During this period, you will lose more pounds. High levels of growth hormone in your body have other health benefits.

Fasting is not famine. Hunger is an involuntary withdrawal of forced food by external forces; This happens in times of war and famine when there is not enough food. Fasting, on the other hand, is voluntary, intentional and dominated. Food is readily accessible, but we choose not to eat it for spiritual, health or other reasons.

Fasting is as old as humanity, much older than any other diet. Ancient civilizations, like the Greeks, recognized that there was something that could be useful for periodic fasting. They were often called healing, purification or detoxification times. Almost all faiths and religions in the world practice fasting rituals.

Before the advent of agriculture, people never took three meals a day plus snacks in between. We ate only when we found food that could be separated for hours or days. Thus, from evolution, three meals a day are not essential for survival. Otherwise, we would not survive as a species.

Towards the 21st century, and we all forget this ancient practice. After all, fasting is bad for business! Food manufacturers encourage us to eat more meals and snacks a day. Nutrition authorities warn that skipping a meal will have serious health consequences. Over time, these messages have very well pierced our heads.

The publication has no standard duration. This can be done for several hours or days before the end of the month. From time to time, fasting is a diet in which we fast to eat regularly. Fasting under 16 to 20 hours is usually done more frequently, even daily. Longer fasts, usually 24 to 36 hours, are done 2 to 3 times a week. It turns out that we all fasted 12 hours between dinner and breakfast.

Millions and millions of people have worked on this publication for thousands of years. Is not it healthy? Many proofs have shown that it has enormous health benefits.

> ## What Happens When We Eat Regularly?

Before enjoying the benefits of intermittent fasting, it is best to understand why taking 5 to 6 meals a day or every six hours (unlike fasting) can do more harm than good.

When we eat, we provide food energy. The essential hormone involved is insulin (produced by the pancreas), which is secreted during the meal. Carbohydrates and proteins stimulate insulin. Fat reduces the effect of insulin, but it is rarely consumed alone.

> ## Insulin has Two Critical Functions:

First, it allows the body to start using food energy immediately. Carbohydrates quickly turn into glucose, increasing blood sugar. Insulin directs glucose to body cells used as energy. The proteins break down into amino acids, and the excess amino acids can be converted to glucose. Protein does not need to increase blood sugar, but it can increase insulin. Fats have a minimal effect on insulin.

Second, insulin stores excess energy for future use. Insulin converts excess glucose into glycogen and stores it in the liver. However, the amount of glycogen stored is limited. When the limit is reached, the liver begins to convert glucose into fat. The fat is deposited in the liver (excess becomes fatty liver) or fatty deposits in the body (often stored as visceral or abdominal fat).

Therefore, when we eat and have breakfast all day long, we are always fed, and our insulin levels remain high. In other words, we can spend most of our day eating food from food.

> **What Happens When We Fast?**
The process of using and storing the food produced when we eat goes the other way when we fast. Insulin levels decrease, which causes the body to start burning stored energy. You first access glycogen, the glucose stored in the liver, and you use it. After that, the body begins to break down the stored body fat into energy.

As a result, the body exists in two states: a condition that feeds on high insulin, and a low insulin voice. We store food energy or burn food energy. If the meal and the fast are balanced, there is no weight gain. If we spend most of our days eating and storing energy, there is a good chance that we will gain weight over time.

> **Intermittent Fasting Versus Continuous Caloric Restriction:**

Strategic calorie control for consistent calorie reduction is the most common dietary recommendation for weight loss and type 2 diabetes. For example, the American Diabetes Association recommends an energy deficit of 500 to 750 kcal/day as well than regular physical activity. Dieters follow this approach and recommend eating between 4 and 6 small meals throughout the day.

Does a long-term portion control strategy work? Rarely! A cohort study in the UK with a follow-up of nine years of 176,495 obese subjects showed that only 3,528 of them had achieved average weight at the end of the study. That's 98% of cancellations.

Intermittent fasting is not a constant caloric restriction. Calorie restriction causes a compensatory increase in hunger and, worse, a decrease in the rate of metabolism in the body, a double curse. Because when you burn fewer calories a day, it is harder to lose weight and after losing it is much easier to recover. This type of diet puts the body in "starvation" mode as the metabolism speeds up to save the energy.

The broken pole has none of these disadvantages.

The benefits of intermittent fasting for health is that it increases metabolism, which leads to weight loss and body fat.

Unlike a daily diet to reduce calories, fasting sometimes increases metabolism. It makes sense from survival. If we do not eat, the body exercise stored energy as fuel to stay alive and find other foods. Hormones allow the body to turn the energy sources of food into body fat.

Studies show this phenomenon. E.g., four days of continuous fasting increased the basal metabolic rate by 12%. The levels of the neurotransmitter norepinephrine, which prepares the body for action, increased by

117%. Fatty acids in the blood increased more than 370% when the body stopped burning food to burning stored fat.

There is no loss of muscle mass.

Unlike a diet with a constant calorie restriction, intermittent fasting does not burn the muscle as much as it fears. In 2010, researchers noted a group of subjects who experienced 70 days of alternate daily fasting (eating a day and fasting the other day). Their muscle mass started at 52.0 kg and ended at 51.9 kg. In other words, there was no muscle loss, but they lost 11.4% fat and found a significant improvement in LDL cholesterol and triglyceride levels.

During fasting, the body naturally brings out more human growth hormone to preserve lean muscles and bones. Muscle mass is usually protected until body fat falls below 4%. As a result, most people are not likely to lose muscle by intermittent fasting.

It cancels insulin resistance, type 2 diabetes and fatty liver.

Type 2 diabetes is a disease characterised by too much sugar in the body, to the point that cells can no longer respond to insulin and absorb more blood glucose (insulin resistance), which leads to the formation of a high blood sugar level. Also, the liver is filled with fat. Eliminate excess glucose by converting it and storing it as fat.

Therefore, to reverse this situation, two things must happen:

- First, stop consuming more sugar in your body.
- Second, burn the remaining sugar.

The best diet to attain this is a diet low in carbohydrates, protein and high in fat also called a ketogenic diet. (Remember that carbohydrates are the richest in blood sugar, with some protein and the least fat). That's why a low carb diet will help you reduce your glucose load. For many people, this is already enough to quell insulin resistance and type 2 diabetes. However, in severe cases, diet is not enough.

What about exercise? Exercise helps to burn glucose in bone muscles, but not in all tissues and organs, including fatty liver. Training is essential, but to eliminate excess glucose in the organs, it is necessary to "cell-out" the cells temporarily.

This can be achieved through occasional fasts. For this reason, historically, people have called post-cleansing or detoxification. It can be a powerful tool to get rid of any excess. This is the fastest way to reduce blood glucose and insulin levels and ultimately reverse insulin resistance, type 2 diabetes and fatso's liver.

Incidentally, taking insulin for type 2 diabetes does not solve the root cause of the problem, namely the excess sugar in the body. Insulin will expel blood sugar, which lowers blood sugar, but where does sugar go? The liver will convert everything into fat, fat in the liver and fat in the stomach. Insulin patients often end up gaining weight, which makes their diabetes worse.

Increases Heart Health.

Over time, high blood glucose levels from type 2 diabetes can damage the blood vessels and nerves that control the heart. The extent a person has diabetes, the more likely they are to develop heart disease. Reducing blood glucose during intermittent fasting also reduces the risk of cardiovascular disease and stroke.

Also, intermittent fasting has been rendering to improve blood pressure, total cholesterol and LDL (bad), blood triglycerides, and markers of inflammation associated with many chronic diseases and increased brain power.

Several trials have shown that fasting has many neurological benefits, including attention and concentration, reaction time, immediate memory, cognition, and the creation of new brain cells. Studies in mice have also shown that intermittent fasting reduces brain inflammation and prevents the symptoms of Alzheimer's disease.

> **What to Expect with the Occasional Publication?**

Hunger Decreases:

Usually, we experience hunger pains almost four hours after a meal. So, if we fast for 24 hrs, does that mean that our hunger will be six times stronger? Of course not.

Many fear that fasting causes extreme hunger and overeating. Studies have shown that the day after a day of fasting resulted in a 20% increase in caloric intake. However, during repeated fasts, hunger and appetite diminish surprisingly.

Hungry in the waves. If we do not do anything, hunger disappears after a while. Drinking tea (of all kinds) or coffee (with or without caffeine) is usually enough to fight it. Nevertheless, it is best to drink it black, because a teaspoon or two of cream or half a half will not cause much reaction to insulin. Do not use any sugar or artificial sweetener. If necessary, a bone broth can also be taken during fasting.

The Blood Sugar does not Deteriorate:

Sometimes people worry that fasting blood sugar will drop sharply during fasting and become shaky and sweaty. This does not happen because the body strictly controls blood sugar, and many mechanisms keep it in the proper range. During fasting, the body starts to break down glycogen in the liver to release glucose. This happens every night during sleep.

If we fast for more than 24 to 36 hours, the glycogen stores are depleted and the liver creates new glucose using glycerol, a by-product of fat breakdown (a process called gluconeogenesis). In addition to using glucose, our brain cells can also use ketones as a source of energy. Ketones are created when fat is metabolized and can provide up to 75% of the energy needs of the brain (the remaining 25% glucose).

The only exception is for people taking diabetes medications and insulin. First, you should consult your doctor because doses may be reduced during fasting. Otherwise, if hypoglycaemia is over treated and develops, which can be dangerous, you need to have some sugar to reverse it. It will quickly break down and make it counterproductive.

The Phenomenon of Dawn:

After fasting, especially in the morning, some people have high blood sugar. This phenomenon of dawn is the result of a circadian rhythm in which, just before waking, the body secretes more elevated levels of various hormones to prepare for the next day:

- Adrenaline: Gives energy to the body.
- Growth Hormone: Repairs and creates a new protein.
- Glucagon: Moves glucose from storage in the liver to the blood for use as energy.
- Cortisol, a stress Hormone: To activate the body.

These hormones peak in the morning and then descend to lower levels throughout the day. In non-diabetic diabetics, the increase in blood sugar is low, and most people do not even realise it. However, most people with diabetes can experience a marked increase in blood sugar levels as the liver is wasting blood sugar.

This will also happen in a long post. When there is no food, insulin levels remain low, while the liver releases some of its stored sugar and fat. It's natural and not bad at all. The strength of the tip will decrease as the organ swells with sugar and fat.

Who should not do a casual job?

- Women who want to become pregnant, are pregnant or breastfeeding.
- Those who are malnourished or overweight.
- Children under 18 years and over.
- Those who have gout.
- People with gastroesophageal reflux disease (GERD).
- People with eating disorders should first consult their doctor.
- People with diabetes and insulin medications should first consult their doctor as doses should be reduced.
- Those taking the medication should first consult their doctor as they may affect the timing of treatment.

- Those who feel very stressed or have problems with cortisol should not fast because fasting is another stressor.
- Those who train on most days of the week should not fast.

How to prepare for a casual job?

If you are preparing to start intermittent fasting, it is best to go on a low carb and high-fat diet for three weeks. This will allow the body to get used to using fats instead of glucose as a source of energy. It means getting rid of all sugars, cereals (bread, cookies, cakes, pasta, rice), legumes and refined vegetable oils. This will minimise most of the side effects associated with fasting.

Start with a message of fewer than 16 hours, for example, from dinner (8 pm) to lunch (noon) the next day. You can usually eat between noon. And 8:00, and you can eat two or three meals. When you feel comfortable with this, you can increase the speed to 18, 20 hours.

Intermittent Fasting for Women

For shorter messages, you can do it daily, continuously. For longer fasts, such as 24 to 36 hours, you can do them 1 to 3 times a week, alternating fasting days and typical meal days.

There is no single fasting mode that is precise. The key is to choose the one that suits you the best. Some people get results with a shorter message, while others may need longer words. Some prepare the classic fast only with water, others make tea and coffee quickly, while others make a quick bone broth. No matter what you do, it's essential to stay hydrated and control yourself. If you do not feel well at any time, stop immediately. You may be hungry, but you should not feel sick.

> **Intermittent Fasting System:**
If you want to reduce a lot of weight, you will have to take a closer look at your diet, but if you're going to lose a few pounds for the beach, you may find that a few weeks of casual fasting can do it for you.

Although there are many different ways, you can do a quick breakneck, and we will only see a smart system running in 24 hours, which I lost weight in two months. The primary method is to fast twice a week for 24 hours. It is, therefore, logical to work several days apart. It's easier to choose a busy day of work, so you do not feel hungry. At first, you will experience hunger pains, but they will pass and, as you get used to intermittent fasting, you may have the hunger that is no longer a problem. You may find that during fasting, you have high concentration, which is the opposite of what you expected, but many feel it.

While you fast, you can and should drink plenty of water to prevent dehydration. Tea and coffee go well while drinking some milk. If you're worried that your body is not getting enough nutrients, think of celery, broccoli, ginger and lime juice, which will taste great and provide a nutrient-rich body. Although if you can handle it, it would be better to keep water, tea and coffee.

Regardless of your diet, whether you are healthy or not, you should notice weight loss after about three weeks of intermittent fasting and do not be discouraged if you do not see much progress at first, this is not a race. It is better to lose weight in a linear fashion in time rather than falling lose a few pounds that you will return directly. After the first month, you may want to examine your fasting diet for several days and eliminate foods high in sugar and unwanted foods that you might otherwise eat. I found that prolonged, intermittent fasting naturally made me want to eat healthier foods.

If you do occasional bodybuilding, you can then examine your macronutrients and calculate the amount of protein and carbohydrate you need to eat, and it's a lot more complicated. You can find information on several websites that you will need to spend time looking for the best results.

The occasional fast has many advantages, which you will notice as you go along; Some of these benefits include more energy, fewer pockets, a clearer mind and a general sense of well-being. It is essential not to be tempted to overeat after fasting, as this will cancel the effect of intermittent fasting.

If you want to lose fat, the intermittent fast is the perfect remedy. Research shows that intermittent fasting that comes and goes during periods of fasting and feeding has tremendous benefits for your body and brain. It can prevent chronic diseases, improve memory and brain function, and increase energy levels. Plus, casual fasting is a potent trick to lose weight quickly without recovering.

Intermittent fasting can speed up your weight loss goals by eliminating stubborn fats, reducing calories and reactivating your metabolism for better performance.

When you fast intermittent, you eat all the food your body needs, but for a shorter period. There are several methods, but the most common is to eat for 6 to 8 hours and the remaining 14 to 16 hours. It's good as it looks, particularly when you add unbreakable coffee to control hunger.

Studies show that intermittent fasting speeds up weight loss. In a 2015 review of 40 different studies, participants weighed an average of 10 books over ten weeks. Another study found that obese adults who occasionally follow the "substitute" supplement program (consuming 25% of their daily calories in a day and often the next day) lost up to 13 pounds in eight weeks.

The success of many diets has also been interrupted: targeting and reducing visceral fat. Visceral fat is stubborn, internal fat that accumulates in the abdominal organs. For six months, people on an intermittent fasting diet could eliminate four to seven per cent of their visceral fat.

> ## How Intermittent Fast Increases Weight Loss Quickly?

If you think about it, the message is not so unnatural. Their ancestors evolved to succeed in situations where food was scarce. In addition to a host of other health benefits, intermittent fasting triggers the perfect storm of metabolic changes to treat weight loss and reduce fat.

➢ **Benefits of Beautiful Fast Include:**

Early-onset of ketosis: As a rule, complete ketosis requires careful planning and extreme restriction of carbohydrates, but intermittent fasting provides direct access to this fat-burning condition. Once your body has exhausted glucose, your primary source of energy, you are forced to burn fat stores for energy as part of a process called ketosis. Ketosis improves the chemistry of your blood, reduces inflammation and helps you lose weight quickly. To burn off excess fat, combine your occasional fast with a Keto diet.

It reduces insulin levels: There are two ways to have an occasional insulin effect. First, it increases adiponectin levels, which helps restore insulin sensitivity to prevent weight gain and diabetes. Second, fasting reduces insulin levels after fasting. Low insulin levels are a signal that your body has to switch to burning stored fat instead of glucose.

Improves cholesterol: A child with intermittent fasting affects cholesterol by lowering LDL and VLDL (bad cholesterol) levels. Although increasing cholesterol does not lead directly to weight loss, overweight and obese people are more likely to have risky high LDL and VLDL cholesterol and cardiovascular risk.

Reducing Inflammation: Reducing inflammation is essential for losing weight, increasing longevity and reducing the risk of serious diseases such as Alzheimer's and cancer. That's why he's at the heart of a safe diet. Occasional fasting reduces oxidative stress and inflammation in all areas, including markers of inflammation such as adiponectin, leptin, and neurotrophic factors derived from the brain.

Increase Metabolism: Intermittent fasting also increases the metabolism of proteins, fats and glucose in animal studies. Increased resting metabolism helps the body burn more calories during the day, even at rest. Fasting also increases the levels of adrenaline and norepinephrine, hormones that help the body release more stored energy (body fat) during fasting.

If you've ever looked for methods to lose weight, you've probably heard the post. But have you heard of casual work? This type of fasting is becoming more and more popular and can have much health benefits in addition to helping to lose weight.

Let's see what a broken message is and how it can help you lose weight. Like any business, it also means refraining from eating for a while. Then follow quickly with a meal in the so-called feeding window. For example, the usual time to fast is 16 hours, followed by an 8-hour control window.

This does not mean that you eat for 8 hours in a row. It merely means that there is a time when you can consume food. Most people opt for two large meals, one breaking the fast and the other an hour before the fast begins. You can also have a snack if you wish, which will occur during the meal period.

One way to make it simple is to include a period of fasting while you sleep. Then you could take your last meal for about 20 hours, then go to bed at any time and eat at noon the next day.

This cycle may be more natural than our current program of three meals a day. Looking at the early years as humans, we ate practically during the day at sunset, then slept after sunset. It was similar to the period after a 16-hour fast, and maybe our body responds well to this fasting system.

> **Is it Healthy for Your Body?**

Intermittent fasting is unlike any other incredible diet since it is a full-sized diet. Many people do not know if this is natural or not. Is it healthy for the body, or can it have effects on the back? We are used to fasting when we are sick or not in the mood and even babies and animals. Therefore, fasting is a natural mechanism that allows the body to stop eating for a while because it has other functions.

Intermittent fasting for weight loss is all about people who want to comply with the actual rules. Eating often with less will allow you to consume all the foods you want, but will inadvertently reduce the number of calories consumed daily. You gain freedom and the ability to lose weight. Intermittent fasting is healthy when you train your body, especially the fasting mechanism. If you provide your body with food the moment your brain tells you that you are hungry, it will reduce appetite. Remember that a starvation mechanism that is alerted every 3-4 hours and three meals a day is not okay to meet the needs of the body equitably. Therefore, an occasional lean weight loss recommends eating six times a day with three small meals and three snacks.

You will be surprised to be satisfied with even half of your usual meal after a few weeks. Wait, and you will notice a reasonable weight loss. Intermittent fasting also has a more significant release of stress hormones. On the contrary, many fall ill when they hear the word quickly because they find this regime very restrictive. Sometimes fasting is not equivalent to a hunger strike. Eating a less rare program is not prohibitive because you can enjoy your favourite foods while reducing your consumption. If you want to eat more of the same food, do it at your next meal.

> **Another Look at the Intermittent Weight Loss Publication:**

Intermittent fasting, or short-term fasting, has turned into a hot topic among people interested in nutrition. It's not a diet in itself, but, a diet. This means that we do not eat more than before and then consume all meals for about eight hours. Does it help people lose weight? It depends mostly on the study you want to believe in and perhaps your own experience.

Major thing to know is that the intermittent fast is not a panacea for weight loss. By importance, people take what they eat, how much they eat, and how much they exercise. But for some people, this can be another valuable tool for losing weight. But we are all awesome people, and there is no way of knowing how it will impact if you try. Like everything else, the best action is to try it and see how things are going.

But this can affect some people for several reasons:

1. Promotes higher sensitivity to insulin. Perhaps because we had to go through periods of celebration and starvation in our genes and our metabolisms are now programmed to work better in the diet and the cycle of hunger. Tests have shown that periods of famine cause an impressive increase in insulin sensitivity.

2. Increased secretion of growth hormone. Somatotropin, the human maturation hormone, increases when we fast. In doing so, somatotropin will promote the breakdown of adipose tissue, the fat that will be used to produce energy when we no longer eat food.

3. It can reduce calorie intake. If you reduce the number of daily meals, you will probably reduce the overall food intake and, consequently, the total number of calories. Of course, this means you will not be satiated for a while.

Energy and hunger are the two most important issues people have or think they have with the occasional fasting program. If you determine to delay or cancel your breakfast and have experienced it in the past, as you may recall, this lack of food resulted in a loss of energy. I can only imagine how hungry and miserable they would be for this first meal of the day. And it could be a moment.

But humans are stuck in a routine, but if we manage to break these habits, we are also very adaptable. This means that if we go through those painful moments when our bodies break from the routines of the past until they adopt a new method, there is a good chance that you will be rewarded. This short period will not hurt a healthy person. However, if a person has difficulty regulating blood sugar, hypoglycaemia or diabetes, they should consult a dietitian or doctor. But for a healthy person, the body takes about 84 hours to fast before the glucose drops to a dangerous level.

> **The Right Way to do it:**

From time to time, fasting or short-term fasting is essential when you drink water only 24 hours out of 2 or 3 times a week. To clarify this, here is an example of a short and fast period.

Monday: Eat regular meals, but do not eat anything else after dinner.

Tuesday: Drink only water all day until dinner. Get a regular meal consisting of healthy foods for this meal. By doing this, you always get the reward of having calories every day.

Before starting this type of fasting, I made sure that missing a meal and not eating for many hours would destroy my metabolism and reduce the muscles I had so hard to gain. However, while reading Brad Pilon's Eat Stop Eat, I discovered that it was a myth and that fasting would have no such effect at that time. However, to be clear, fasting longer than that or following a very low-calorie diet for weeks will result in a slower metabolism, so do not go.

The diet has fewer calories.

When you look at one form of the diet, it's just a method of consuming fewer calories and consuming more than eating.

This is the essential guideline of any weight reduction, and it will never change. If you

Intermittent Fasting for Women

follow the diet entirely without cheating, you will lose weight; however, it is merely a matter of asking the right method to follow.

That's why I believe that intermittent fasting once or twice a week is the solution to lose weight quickly. It's easy to follow as it does not require too much planning and organisation, and I found that I was saving money because I ate less.

But the main reason I think it works so well is that it does not look like a diet. Of course, the days of fasting may be a little tight, but the more they work, the more comfortable they are, and you always know that you are going to eat that day. Also, on fasting days, you can still eat whatever you want within reasonable limits. Of course, if you continue to eat a lot of junk food, your results will not be as good. But I have found that a healthy and regular diet, including a weird meal can quickly lose fat and maintain it without real effort.

I believe that casual fasting is a healthy and correct way to lose weight fast. It allows you to reduce your calorie intake quickly and, as a result, create a significant deficit, crucial for successful weight loss.

> **A Fantastic Secret on Weight Loss:**

Fasting is an act of refraining from food and drink. Absolute fast is far from food and drink. The fasting juice will stay away from food but will drink milk and other liquids. Fasting is sometimes another problem.

Most people who plan fast to lose weight. They have the idea that eating a small amount of food and that hunger will make a body leaner and more fit. Yes, for practical and logical reasons, you can lose weight because small amounts of food mean losing weight. But what was behind this logical reasoning was the scientific explanation behind these weight loss effects.

There are also practical statements that show the effects of fasting. But can fasting lose weight?

Yes, at some point, starving can make you thinner, which is because in the absence of water and once hydrated, you will recover this more massive body. So it's just a waste of time.

There are also scientific explanations that starve and make the body adapt. Once you consume food, the body will store fat in reserve. This means that your body will have poor metabolism once you are hungry. Then a weight loss job will not do you any good.

We must remember that experts do not recommend the staff. Always remember that there is no easy way to get good results and that it's the same as losing weight. You must also strive to achieve your goals.

Staying healthy but fit means combining healthy eating with proper exercise and a healthy mind-set. Also, avoid stress and other psychological factors.

> Here are some Applicative Ways to Lose Weight:

Eating often, but in small amounts, will allow the body to eat small amounts of food. In the long term, our body will adapt to lower amounts of food but will not store fat as a carrier.

Drinking water before each meal will result in small amounts of food that you consume.

Exercise of weight loss (obviously?).

Staying out of the calories you need every day is a great idea. You can find out by multiplying your weight (in pounds) by 18.

Stay away from too much carbohydrate and fat-based foods. Choose foods that are high in protein.

Conventional wisdom holds that you need to eat less and exercise more to lose weight. As a result, more and more people are on a low-calorie diet to lose weight. Many people now even quickly lose weight. But there is a good and a wrong way to fast, and most people do it poorly.

> **A Shocking Study:**
In the 1940s, scientist Ancel Keys conducted the most extensive research on hunger. He took 40 healthy men and put them at 1600 calories a day for three months to observe the effects of caloric restriction.

He had good news for those who were interested in fasting to lose weight. Participants lost 25% of their initial weight, but they were afraid of them.

Participants complained that they were cold, tired and hungry all the time. They felt dizzy and could not concentrate. They were too old and lose interest in sex. They have even become depressed and worried.

Remember, it was 1600 calories a day, which is more than most health authorities recommend to consume now if you are trying to lose weight, can you imagine what would happen if you tried to fast?

➢ **Best Way to Fast:**
Traditionally, fasting is staying hungry without eating or with very little food. As I said, not only will you lose fat, but you will also lose muscle, destroy your metabolism and increase your vulnerability to mental illness.

Fortunately, there is a better way to lose weight on an empty stomach. This method uses only short periods of fasting, cyclic periods with complete feeding and is called intermittent fasting.

It has been found that occasional fasting burns fat but does not burn muscles. Also, it is much easier to skip a meal or two than to skip some meals or cut them when you eat, and you are still hungry.

If that was not enough, it was found that occasional fasting reduced the risks of diabetes, cancer and heart disease.

➤ Apply the Occasional Fast to Your Life:

So, how can I start with the occasional publication? There are several ways: you have to start by skipping breakfast one day. Was it hard for you? Continue to skip breakfast as much as possible until you do it straight for five days.

Now you have options. You can continue by skipping breakfast every day or skipping lunch one day a week. Either way, you will turn your body into a machine to develop your muscles.

➤ Tips to be Sure when You Publish a Weight Loss:

Fasting weight loss is a safe weight loss technique if you maintain a quick will, but this can be dangerous if you work too hard or improperly. Fasting to lose weight can cause organic damage, loss of muscle mass and heart attack. So, if you are reasoning of fasting to lose weight, a three-day fast is the best thing to do, and you should use the following safety precautions.

➢ Quick Post Tips.

1. Never drink water fast. This can expel the necessary chemicals from your body and cause complications due to an irregular heartbeat and complete heart failure. Fasting this way is not wise.

2. They must be supervised by a certified health professional and not just use the new age digital book as a smart guide. Post weight loss should be made properly.

3. Do not chew gum or other substances in the mail. Chewing tells the stomach to start producing acid for digestion. Consume it until it loses weight, which can cause heartburn.

4. It took years for the body to be restored; So it's not about what you want it to be overnight.

Safe Fasting Methods.

Of course, a three-day fast is not the only way to fast. You can start with the occasional fasting method in which you fast every other day and usually eat in the middle. This is belike a safer way to do it, but remember, do not just be quick with water, follow the established guidelines. The fast-food guide, Eat, Stop, Eat, describes a safe program for occasional fasting for fat loss.

Fasting can take many forms, which does not mean that you do not always eat food. For example, you can go to a part-time job where you only eat vegetables or fruit. This weight-loss item could be the safest method to achieve fasting, and it is helpful to reduce weight.

Jon Benson, as part of his fast-food guide, Diet Every Other Day, has created a different and effective dietary program. This simple system is in its second version and uses the SNAPP feeding process to guide the child through a weight loss system allowing him to eat without dieting every other day. This meal regales you with your favourite foods, which motivates you to continue the process.

So, if you plan to fast to lose weight, be sure to do it safely and effectively. If you choose to do it carefully, you will look much thinner and healthier.

➤ **It Works Well if Done Like This:**

Fasting or to stop eating is not a way to lose weight properly. We all need a certain amount of nutrition each day to maintain a healthy metabolism and immune system. Depriving the body of one of these essential components of biochemistry means risking one's life in the name of losing weight.

Some celebrities claim to have been on a detox diet where they only drank water and fibre to clean their impurity system. The only scientific proof is that they have lost weight. Here we consider fasting as a way to lose weight and nothing else. So how fast can we lose weight properly?

It is not healthy to miss food altogether for the reasons outlined above. Your body has specific nutritional needs, especially vitamins and plant-based chemicals (photochemical) that support your immune system and your metabolism. Without this, you can become extremely sick.

Also, the argument that by consuming only liquid foods without solids, our body will be forced to burn fat does not hold water. All the beneficial components of our diet are reduced in water and fat-soluble liquids. What drives your body to burn fat is the lack of carbs in your diet, not the absence of solid foods. However, by incorporating enough fruit and vegetable juices into your liquid diet and drinking about three litres of purified water each day, you need to lose weight and continue to consume enough nutrients to maintain critical biochemical processes in your body.

Preparing for such a publication will help your body get the most out of it. Some claim that colon cleansing will help reduce the effects of digestive problems, although this can be discussed. However, it will not hurt, so if you think it will help you, it could give you a psychological boost.

Also, before fasting, you do not need to replenish carbohydrates as this will delay or even prevent weight loss. This is not how you should lose weight properly. A quick weight loss should also be a healthy weight loss. It is neither healthy nor sensible to feed before fasting.

Fasting is not complete either, and nothing is taken orally except perhaps water. This could damage your system by unnecessarily depriving you of nutrition. Consider your reason for fasting: losing weight. The most effective method to decrease weight quick isn't to eat, yet to compel your body to utilize fat as a wellspring of vitality to fuel your digestion. You should be able to do this while maintaining a sufficient diet to avoid permanent or long-term damage to the immune system or any other bodily process.

So how should you publish in a healthy enough way to achieve this? You should first consider your daily routine. You should not fast if you do not avoid hard work or situations that could be dangerous if you feel weak. Fasting affects some people in this way, and you do not have to fast during your period.

Decide if you intend to fast for an extended period of only two or three days at a time, with a feeding period in between. If this is the last case, how should your diet be between periods of fasting? Some associate fast-casual fast with juice, so that at least they take diets, but again, you have to be careful not to jeopardise your basic bodily processes. Your liver needs some degree of nutrition to stay functional.

If you are not utilised to fasting, it will be difficult to stay without food for more than a day, but that's all you need. If you fast from dawn to dawn the next morning, it will not only give your digestive system a well-deserved rest that will benefit you, but it will also form the basis of a healthy weight loss program that will not compromise your well-being. Here's how you need to lose weight properly.

Doing this two or three times a month will reduce the effects of prolonged fasting on your body and will also help eliminate many of the toxins accumulated in your system. When you stop quickly, first drink two glasses of salted lemon water to rinse the order, then have your breakfast as usual.

➤ **Show Weight Loss is Extremely Effective:**

Fasting has a bad reputation as a diet plan. You see, many believe that your metabolism will slow down if you do not eat every few hours.

The idea of "slowing down your metabolism" is the biggest myth of the fitness industry. Your metabolic diet may slow down with a chronic, hard and low-calorie diet, but for weeks and weeks, there is a constant restriction of calories.

A study on people who lose body fat on a diet of 800 calories a day (American College of Nutrition 1999):

1. They took 20 people on a daily diet of 800 calories.

2. Ten people underwent cardiovascular training three times a week.

3. Ten people practised resistance three times a week.

Results: No muscle loss in the resistance group and higher resting metabolism than before onset. Thus, even with a diet of 800 calories a day, the metabolism did not slow down (as long as resistance exercise was practised several times a week).

Resistance training is the key to losing weight during aggressive dieting.

What is the connection with fasting?

The publication I recommend is called an informal notification.

1. Eat regularly until dinner (2 to 4 meals as usual).

2. Stop eating after dinner.

3. Fast until dinner the next day.

4. Eat your usual dinner for this meal.

This allows a 24-hour fast and still has few calories throughout the day. The approach I teach is to work up to 2-3 times a week.

Your body rarely stores carbohydrates in the form of fat to a significant degree.

Almost all the fat you see in your body comes from the fat you eat.

CHAPTER THREE

Intermittent Weight Loss:

➢ Pros and Cons:
Weight loss, help with the cellular repair process, improving mental health and transparency, and reducing insulin resistance are the main benefits of intermittent fasting for women.

➢ **Weight Loss:**
The most common reason people have for considering intermittent fasting is perhaps the reduction in the number of food they eat, as well as their overall caloric intake.

Although I do not follow the intermittent lifestyle to lose weight, eating regular meals for a short time makes you feel full almost all day long. As a result, most people are bored of not grazing.

After 12 hours, your body enters a state called "fasting". On an empty stomach, your body can burn inaccessible fats during a meal.

When we enter the fasting state only 12 hours after the last meal, our body is rarely in this state of fat burning. This is one of the rationality why many people who start fasting sometimes lose fat without changing their diet or exercise frequency. Fasting can cause your body to burn fat, which rarely occurs during a healthy meal.

➤ **Consider All Repair Procedures:**
"Sleep heals everything," said my grandmother. And of course, that's the message.

When you sleep, your body start to repair its cells and perform its hormonal cycles. And when your body does not have to digest, it can focus entirely on the cellular repair process.

Cell repair, also called autophagy, is a process in which cells begin to eliminate waste and repair themselves. This procedure is necessary to maintain muscle mass and reduce the undesirable effects of ageing. Autophagy = fountain of youth. Ok, a little exaggerated, but you understand!

When you fast, your body can perform its repair and healing work. There is much research that fasting can help the process of cell renewal in cancer and other diseases.

> **Increasing Mental Health and Insurance:**

Without a doubt, one of my favourite benefits of the occasional fast is the mental clarity I have in the morning.

It can take five to seven hours to think about homework and a lot of work in that window. After starting to eat, I am less focused and a little slower. My afternoon at the office is less productive.

Coincidentally, non-digestible coffee has two benefits: mental clarity and concentration. Combined with fasting, I often feel unstoppable at work.

> **Reduce the Insulin Resistance:**

Insulin resistance occurs when our body does not respond to insulin as it should and cannot easily absorb blood sugar. This is often due to poor nutrition, genetics, inactivity, high blood pressure, overweight or obesity. It is said that occasional hunger reduces insulin resistance.

In other words, when your body can not properly break down blood glucose, it starts to store it as fat. Intermittent fasting helps to restore blood sugar, which brings us to our next random number for women.

➢ **It Remains Difficult for a Long Time:** Fasting requires that you spend a specified period without eating at all, and that you eat a certain amount of calories over some time and that you repeat it to create a calorie deficit. This long period of calorie-free eating can be challenging to maintain in the long-term because of the low energy, cravings, habits, and discipline needed to meet the specific time frames of your fasting periods.

Sometimes fasting is also difficult to maintain in the long run because of the amount of self-control needed to do it. Both sides of the casual post can be steep; do not eat when you have to fast, and overeating at the time of eating is just as important.

Brad Pilon, researcher and author of "Eat, Stop, Eat," suggests, "Once your message is over, you should pretend never to be fast - no compensation, no reward, no special diet, no cherries, no drink, no special pill.".

While this may be difficult to do, it is crucial for the process and ultimately, reap the benefits of intermittent fasting.

➤ Weigh or no Weigh?

If you are planning to lose weight like most people these days, you may feel a little attached to the scale of your bathroom. However, there is a better "weight", sorry for fullness, to control the progress of weight loss than relying on this "irrelevant" and outdated method.

It's you when the number on the scale goes down, you're shouting with joy and accomplishment, but when that number goes up, you feel defeated and wondering what the benefit is actually? If so, it is unfortunate that "weight" is not what you should consider to measure your results and the feeling of defeat serves only to discourage you from additional efforts to lose weight.

"Weighing" is the least effective way to measure your health and your progress. Scale measurements are the amount of blood in your body, the undigested food in your digestive system, the fluid in your lymphatic system, the glycogen in the liver, muscles and other body components that can fluctuate during the day and from day today.

It is quite reasonable that the amount of fluid in the body fluctuates. Water represents more than 60% of the total weight of the body. However, the extra weight reflected on the scale as water retention is often amenable for the opinion of failure felt by those trying to lose weight. Although water retention is average, a large amount of water retention can be prevented. Ironically, the lack of water and liquids contributes to water retention. Dieters often limit not only calories but also fluid intake. This may be because they skip the caloric drinks less substitute them with water when the body is divested of water, they observe it as a threat to their survival and compensates for it by

Intermittent Fasting for Women

conserving water. Also, if the diet contains too much sodium (as in many American diets), the body still retains more water. Drinking enough water will help you maintain proper water balance and eliminate excess sodium. A right amount of water varies from person to person, but it is generally recommended to drink ounces per kilogram of body weight.

A common cause of water retention in women occurs just before menstruation and almost always disappears as quickly as it appears. Again, you can reduce weight gain by drinking plenty of water, avoiding high-sodium-rich foods, and maintaining an exercise program.

Another component of the body that can balance is the amount of glycogen or carbohydrate stored by the body. The body stores carbohydrates in the liver and muscles, in the form of glycogen. This backup is crucial when you cannot eat, for example, when you sleep or when you bring a lot of energy quickly and unexpectedly. This reserve of energy (glycogen stores or carbohydrates) weighs about a kilogram and is combined with 3 to 4 kilograms of water, hence the word "carbohydrates". Unless you consume the refined carbs (as many do when you start an unhealthy diet), your glycogen stores will be drained and thus the water it contains. However, the body cannot spend a lot of time without proper carbohydrates. Therefore, when the body renews its reserve of carbohydrates, the associated water returns. Do not worry about weight changes up to 2 pounds per day, even without changing your calorie intake or energy expenditure. This is completely normal and has nothing to do with fat loss. Unfortunately, the worst this creates is to create anxiety when the scale is not going in the desired direction.

Remember the real weight of the food you eat. If you have just eaten dinner and the food has not been digested, you can carry a lot of marbles because the food and drinks you have only just consumed can weigh 4 pounds. It is not a weight gain. The message here is that it does not weigh immediately after eating, because the extra weight is the weight of the food. Instead, start by weighing in the morning before eating food or drinks, but remember that the morning weight is not representative of what we are looking for because we are dehydrated in the morning. The first thing to do when waking up is to drink water.

If you are still not convinced that the weight gain of 4 pounds that you managed to take after dinner does not represent the weight of food, consider this: to save 1 pound of fat, you must burn off 3,500 calories. If the 4 pounds you acquire from your dinner were stored as fat, it would mean eating 14,000 calories, which is neither likely nor humanly possible. The same reasoning can go in a different direction. To lose pounds of fat, you need to reduce your intake or increase your activity by 3,500 calories. A weight loss of only 1 to 2 pounds per week is realistic, but if you were on a very low-calorie diet and lost 10 pounds in a week, that weight loss was not due to fat loss, but weight loss of water, glycogen or muscle. Ten pounds of weight loss per week would be equivalent to a reduction of 35,000 calories this week. Does this make sense?

Also to water, glycogen stores undigested food in the gastrointestinal tract, some of the weight is muscle, bone, glycogen stores, organs and fat. Therefore, if you lose weight, we lose some of these ingredients. The reality is that the scale cannot tell us how much of the weight we lost. Unfortunately, what often happens when people opt for the wrong kind of diet is that they do not always lose fat, but lose valuable active muscle mass, which ultimately helps reduce fat loss and future difficulties. To maintain a healthy weight A professional, like a licensed dietitian, to lose weight the right way and start using the right measurement tool to determine success. One of these measurement tools is one that measures "body composition" to give you a percentage of your body's muscle tissue, as well as body fat.

In addition to determining the composition of your body through simple tests, what is the best tool to measure the success of your weight loss? You may be surprised, but the best tool for measuring weight is a mirror. Do you look healthier? Are you less inflated? The second best tool for measuring weight are your feelings. Your feelings are never guilty. You feel better? Do you think your clothes are better? Are the rings getting loose on the fingers? Are your muscles tense? And the third-best tool for measuring weight is a change in your lifestyle? If you do the right things most of the time, you will get the results you are looking for. If you eat correctly, exercise, sleep well and control your stress, do not let the small, normal fluctuations of the scales tell you the opposite.

Let's face it, and even if we are armed with all this knowledge about what constitutes our body weight, it will always be difficult for us humans to leave the scales. So, if you have to use a variety, some experts advise against weighing yourself at least two months after starting a new lifestyle to adapt your body to your unique style. And again, humans enjoy immediate pleasure. So, if you insist on regret, you only do it once a week, preferably at the same time of the day. The morning after waking is usually the best time of the day because we tend to lose less.

But do not forget this figure on the scale is not the sum of your success.

➤ **Reasons Why You Should Throw the Scale:**

The alarm is ringing. It is at 6 o'clock. The old saying that "delay the thief of time" comes to mind. He feels the need to sleep a bit more but gets out of bed crawling.

You go directly to the bathroom. But first, you want to know your weight. Your fitness specialist recommends that you gain weight regularly. When you enter the scale, you notice that the wheel has not changed since the last time you weighed five days ago. You check at your image in the mirror. You do not like what you see. Belly fat seems to have increased. Enthusiastic and disappointed, you go to the bathroom. Are you aware of this scenario? Here are some tips to help you succeed in your quest to lose weight.

You must understand that you are where you are because of your actions. In your turn, your efforts are the result of your reflection. Instead of focusing on your size, be determined to change your thinking and therefore, your actions. Part of the problem comes from your balance. here's why.

1. We gain weight for a long time a few kilos a year, often from 30 years old. From time to time, we eat and lose a few pounds to earn them with interest. Many times, the scale does not reveal subtle changes.

2. When you exercise and do everything you can but cannot see the small changes on the scale, you find yourself unable to do anything. The slaughterhouse of failure becomes your destiny.

3. Balance makes the law of cause and effect forget. Weight gain is an effect, not a cause. The reason is elsewhere: it can be your diet, lack of exercise or a medical problem.

4. Balance can be an excuse for not taking responsibility for your bad eating habits. When you do everything you can and do not see a large resize, you can start to blame the scale, which is defective. That is true. A bad worker blames his tools.

5. Keeping running of what you eat is the key to winning the fight to lose weight. Some experts recommend keeping track of your track record rather than keeping track of what you are spending. Unfortunately, this action deceives your subconscious by telling you that you are acting and that you are healthier. But the truth is that you are worse.

To what extent are weight loss challenges practical and motivating to all members of your group?

Weight loss can be a fun and motivating way to lose weight. If you want to take on a weight loss challenge, try the following:

Gather the group. You must have at least three people to take on the challenge of losing weight in a fun and exciting way. The correct group number would be ten people. In this way, people can come together to help each other. With too few or too many people, participants can quickly leave.

➢ **Good Reward:**
Although losing weight is a great reward, we will never succeed until we succeed. The

best way to incite everyone is to love the title everyone would like to win. Ideas can include money, gifts, vacations, etc. Divide the prize by everyone participating in the challenge, and the winner wins all the awards.

➢ **Use the Percentage of Weight Loss:**
The best way to see who has gained weight is to watch your weight loss percentage. Initially, everyone should stick to the same clothes at the same time. At the end of the competition, you must do the same and then determine the weight loss percentage for each person. Whoever has the highest loss rate will win. E.g.:

At the start of the challenge, Jen weighs 180, Pat weighs 225 and Tom 250, and at the end of the challenge, Jen weighs 140, Pat weighs 190 and Tom 200.

Here is a formula used to see who wins:

Jen $140/180 = 0.777$

Pat $190/225 = .844$

Volume $200/250 = .8$

That means Jen weighs 77% of what she used before. As a result, she lost 23%. (100-77 = 23)

Pat lost 16% (100-84 = 16)

Tom lost 20% (100-80 = 20)

As you can see, Jen has won a significant percentage of her weight loss.

The last tip I would like to give you regarding the challenge of weight loss is to set a time limit for the problem. Some weeks will be too short to change weight, and you will not enjoy all the benefits of such a fast-paced lifestyle. I would recommend that you work for 2-3 months. This will give you a lot of time to lose weight, but it will not be too dull for any of the participants.

➢ **Science on Benefits of Intermittent Fasting:**

Scientists have discovered many benefits of intermittent fasting that, for one reason or another, one must limit caloric intake. Intermittent consumption of about fifteen hours is sometimes described. With this technique, many features of the body can be modified for the better. The real question is not whether fasting can or not, but how it will help you and how often you should do it.

This fasting style has been shown to lower blood pressure and increase HDL levels. This can significantly help control diabetes and can also help you lose weight. All these effects sound pretty good and can be achieved with this type of message. Studies on different kinds of animals show that limiting their calorie consumption increases their lifespan by up to 30%.

Studies in humans have shown that it lowers blood pressure, blood glucose, and insulin sensitivity. With these tests, it is logical to think that fasting, if done for a long time, will increase the life span. The same results can be achieved by cutting calories by 30% all the time, but it has been shown to cause depression and irritability. Fasting is a solution that comes instead of just reducing calories and benefits without depression or irritability.

Intermittent fasting works by eating food every other day. During the days you eat, you end up eating almost double of what you would eat otherwise. You still get an equal number of calories, but you also get all the benefits. This will reduce your stress level and improve your overall health level. This type of fasting is a great way to achieve better fitness, live longer and feel better all the time.

Everyone still wonders what the next big secret of the food industry is. In particular, people want to burn fat and build muscles by investing as little as possible. They want everything, and sometimes it takes too much, at least in most programs.

But what if I told you that the programs that can be used for this, are offered to the entire industry? Enter the occasional publication.

We destroy the highly humanized myth before turning to the benefits of occasional fasting.

Breakfast is the most essential meal of the day:

This myth is quickly killed. Those who regularly fast (often sleeping from breakfast, which means skipping breakfast) report increased concentration, higher energy levels, and a better mood during fasting. Looking for a new coffee? You have found one that burns fat and gives you energy.

Eating six meals a day speeds up your metabolism:

If you consume the same amount of calories and have the equal distribution of macronutrients (we are talking mainly about protein), consume these calories and nutrients between 6 servings and a difference close to 0. Because at the end of the day with one If I reduced calories, the same caloric deficit would occur and if I added calories, it would lead to an equivalent excess.

And if there is a difference, I tend to believe that it is in favour of the publication.

By increasing your sensitivity to insulin, an occasional fast can help you reach your muscles directly when you eat calories, and when you're not fasting, the adrenaline/norepinephrine boost will give you energy and burn fat.

So, what is an intermittent publication?

In the purest sense, intermittent fasting is between the feeding period and the non-feeding period. I will describe the benefits below. However, the general reason for intermittent fasting (IF) participation is that many people respond to the consumption of most of their calories in a small meal, especially during a diet.

This allows you to control hunger, insulin sensitivity (read muscle building) and more time to burn fat (increased adrenaline/norepinephrine).

You can go to bedfast in the afternoon and then eat food a few hours. I would also like to exercise during this period.

Or it may mean getting up and eating a meal and being late in the day until the second/last lunch.

Be smart and efficient. Select a program that will provide results using the effective methods explored. In both cases, you take responsibility for your free time, but for the best results, choose, analyse and listen to your body.

Possible benefits of Intermittent Fasting:

- An increase in insulin sensitivity and secretion of nutrients is a great way to develop muscles without fat accumulation.
- Increased adrenaline/norepinephrine, which means more time to burn fat.
- Reduces appetite and hunger, the ability to feel full due to the consumption of all the calories in fewer meals.
- Increase in energy and concentration.

For example:

If you had 1800 calories in your diet, would you rather eat 2,900 calories or 6,300 calories?

That's all you want in your diet. We want to reap all the benefits when we build the body of our dreams, and this is the ideal way to do it. Here's how you reach your number one goal in the fitness industry: burn fat while building muscles.

Small Detection:

Sometimes the publication is ahead of the rest of the industry. This goes against many of the central myths in the process of initiation that you can believe. But again, we have to ask ourselves if we want the main results. Or do we want to be above average, unique and exaggerated? Be my answer.

> Clenbuterol:

One of the fastest frustrations a person can have is not being able to lose weight immediately. It is not uncommon to hear several people complaining that losing weight for them is the task of Sisyphus, who, according to the Greek myth, would have been condemned to the underworld for throwing stones on a hill, only to discover that they would roll then.

Like Sisyphus, those who are trying to lose weight must always face the intense frustration that even when they have succeeded, something has happened; They start gaining weight again. Like a rock that has been pushed upward, so have the weights that were previously bred. You can imagine the frustration so close to what you were trying to do, to make your efforts useless.

For some people, this could be a problem of discipline: discipline to continue to exercise, training to eat only the right foods and the desire not to eat foods in quantities that can only contribute to the taking of food. Weight. However, even when people adhere to a strict diet designed to achieve an optimal loss of profit, some people are still trying to stop losing weight.

When this happens, it probably means that you have problems with the wrong dietary supplements that you use. If this is the reason, you should start thinking twice before continuing with your current supplement and finding a new one. Fortunately, there is a new supplement that can update and improve your weight loss diet.

This medicine is what people call "clen". This is an abbreviation of the generic name

Clenbuterol. What is this supplement for, and how does it contribute to optimal weight loss for a person?

➤ What is Clenbuterol?

Clenbuterol is a bronchodilator. The main indication of treatment is for people with bronchial asthma. Its main effect on the body is to reduce the obstruction of the human airways to facilitate the breathing of people with these conditions. The effect of Clenbuterol is also durable.

However, in addition to being a bronchodilator, Clenbuterol has other effects on your body. It usually increases the body's muscle mass, which thins the body by reducing the amount of fat that a person has. The primary users of Clenbuterol are athletes and bodybuilders who wish to keep a slim and muscular body.

➤ Clenbuterol is Good for Losing Weight:

You can now see that this medicine is a miracle that you have been looking for all those years in which you tried to lose weight. Clenbuterol is ideal for your weight loss diet and should be taken with the regular food and exercises that you work with. With your ability to increase the size of your muscles and reduce fat at the same time, you can do more than just losing weight. You can also have a statue that can make people envy your success.

> **Time to Time Benefits:**

A diet called "Intermittent Fasting" usually means a shift for a while and a snack for a while. Many choose a 24-hour fast cycle, then eat healthy the next day and continue this process as a lifestyle change.

Animal research has been conducted to determine the benefits of this type of fasting, and you will be happy to know that this can be beneficial to your health.

From time to time, fasting can add 40% to 56% more years to your life. That's just reason enough to do it. However, weight loss and fat oxidation are other benefits.

When you fast, your body is forced to purify the fuel, eliminating old and damaged cells. This cleans up the collection of unwanted things and helps with weight loss and the benefits of choosing the right foods to increase and have a more beneficial effect on your body.

It has been shown that rats are long-term and have improved their survival after heart failure after following an adult diet plan. The researchers also said it could help fight age-related cognitive deficits, so it tells me that it could help prevent Alzheimer's and other types of dementia.

The risk of heart disease and other heart diseases can also be reduced when a healthy, intermittent fasting diet begins. Your risk of other diseases and chronic conditions is likely to be reduced.

You can start healthier with occasional fasts and healthy food choices. Keep carbohydrates up to 50-100 grams daily. Many women eat between 1,200 and 1,500 calories a day, and when they limit their carbs, they continue to lose weight. Men can manage up to 2000 calories a day. Of course, the least is the best, and you need to determine your caloric intake based on your activity, such as work and exercise.

Drink lots of fluids, especially water, and exercise in the evening if possible. This will help with those night cravings.

Once you start eating and drinking healthier, your body will not want to eat junk food (if you have one), so the decision to eat healthy will become more enjoyable as you go through the routine intermittent fasting.

Alternatively, fast daily or ADF means alternate days of eating without eating. However, there is also an intermittent publication called Modified Publication, in which you consume about 20% of your average number of calories a day, then eat normally (but healthy) the next day. This is often more accessible to people because they feel less disadvantaged when they can at least eat something every day while enjoying the majority of the benefits of an ADF diet.

No matter of what you decide to do, be sure to tell your health care provider about your plans so that he or she knows and can work with you to achieve your goals. If you want to lose weight, lose it and feel better, casual fasting can be the solution for you.

Intermittent fasting, or short, is not a process of eating or fasting. It's a diet. When you fast and reduce your caloric intake, you can lead a healthier and longer life. Remember that our ancestors were collectors and hunters. They did not eat all the time, and what they ate was based on what was available. That being said, our bodies are also designed to spend many hours without eating. You can survive without three meals a day and live if life has many benefits that will be explained below.

➢ **Health Benefits:**

1. You remain complete. Some think that fasting or dieting is the same thing as starving. However, during intermittent fasting, ghrelin, a hormone that indicates hunger, adapts to a new way of eating the body so that you do not feel hungry.

2. They will have better access and concentration. Once on an empty stomach, more catecholamine's are produced, which is another hormone in the body. The result is

that you will be more focused on what you do.

3. You will have more power. Because you will not eat as much, there will be less hesitation in blood sugar levels. This means that the real power will be more consistent. Also, the risk of diabetes is reduced. You can also exercise it during exercise, which will increase your body's potential to burn more fat. Growth hormone increases during fasting, which helps burn calories.

4. Burn more fat, which means losing weight. If you eat less and consume fewer calories, your body will become an adipose organ that burns energy instead of taking power from foods you eat regularly if you do not fast. It also means that your body will show more lean muscle mass. On the other hand, if you are starving for about 16 hours, your body is already consuming body fat.

5. You can also use the following items:

• Less blood sugar and better insulin levels.

• Less inflammation.

• Protection against diseases such as heart disease, Alzheimer's disease, and cancer.

➢ How to Start:

Its recommended before looking for a job, you should seek the help of a professional. However, you can start by choosing a day to skip breakfast. You can want to drink water or tea instead of breakfast. As you go, try to go further by skipping lunch. If you feel that you need to eat or are anxious, you can eat a regular size meal.

From time to time, fasting is a new feeding method that has received a lot of attention lately. Everyone tells us that to lose weight, and you have to exercise regularly and with high intensity. While regular exercise is essential for maintaining health and burning fat, the question is "is exercise enough?"

In my opinion, no. Without a change of diet, it is virtually impossible to lose weight and stay away from it all the time. This is where most people move away from diet and exercise because, according to conventional wisdom, you have to lose the food you love, to lose weight.

But what if you do not do it?

Breaking weight loss is not necessarily a new concept. In many cultures, fasting is part of life for cultural and religious reasons. In these cases, fasting is not about losing weight, but about cleaning the body. At times, this method of fasting lasts from a few days to a month.

What happens if instead of fasting for days, we fast every day? The occasional weight loss methods do just that. Instead of fasting for days or weeks, an IF (intermittent fasting) doctor fasts daily, at 4 pm.

A typical day of daily meals for most people is:

8:00 am breakfast.

Lunch.

19:00 dinner.

Maybe a snack before bedtime.

This schedule means that the food is divided into a window to eat for over 12 hours, allowing you to overeat.

Intermittent fasting permits you to eat relatively the same amount of food, only in a short period. An occasional weight loss program would look like this:

10:00 breakfast.

14:00 lunch.

18:00 dinner.

What we did is press the meal window for 8 hours. Outside the 8-hour window, only water should be consumed. These have several significant advantages. For starters, you'll eat less food because most people do not digest food fast enough to consume the same amount of food as in a larger feed window.

Eating less food and consuming the same daily effort will be equivalent to losing weight. Also, as your water intake increases, your body has more opportunities to eliminate excess sodium and waste.

Does fasting work sometimes? I used it to release fat while maintaining muscle and strength. There is a period of mental adjustment of about two weeks. It is a period that usually causes your body and mind to become accustomed to dietary changes.

After two weeks, hunger begins to decline.

> **Amazing Truths about Intermittent Fasting:**

1. You will not feel as hungry as you think. I found that I did not know about food any more than I usually think. When I tried for the first time, I was a little suspicious, but I found it comfortable.

2. Your level of concentration will improve considerably. If I have to do a particularly unique job, I keep it for one of my fastest days because I know I can focus much more effectively on this job.

3. Save money. This is an obvious benefit. You do not pay for the food you do not eat. When I ate six small meals a day, I had to go shopping to organize all my food for the week. Thank God, I'm free of it now!

4. The weight will fall like crazy. I was shocked at how quickly they removed the extra pounds and continue to lose weight. The last two months have included Christmas, and I love food & drinks, and I

always go out thinner than when I walked in. Rapid weight loss is a formality.

5. You will feel happier. You are on the path of the body you deserve and every week, that passes, will show you the progress you are making. It's both motivating and encouraging.

6. Nothing else in your life needs change. This is a typical Sunday for me: a bacon sandwich for breakfast, two pints at lunch, a roast lamb/veal dinner, a few glasses of wine and, in the evening, a light bite. I have been doing this every Sunday since I started the casual job to remind myself that I can and must always enjoy the pleasures of life.

7. You have more time. I realized that during fasting days, I have at least an hour of productive overtime just because I do not cook, cook, or clean.

8. Olympic dream. I sleep like a baby during my fasting days, probably because I'm not so full of food.

9. Much more energy. I feel ten years younger. It may be because I am much

lighter, but it may be because my blood glucose is better regulated, which is a beneficial side effect of intermittent fasting.

10. Eating decreases en masse. I seem to have lost my hope to eat fries, snacks and other minefields diet. It is as if the occasional fast had restored the way you eat.

11. You can gain it as a part of your life, overnight. When I finished my second job, I knew that I could sometimes fast as part of my routine. In doing so, the much-desired weight loss will occur automatically.

12. No small dishes or bars. I cannot make all the smoothies and snacks that the big diet companies think I will satisfy. I want to eat real food in reasonable portions.

13. Eat when you want. You do not eat breakfast, do not worry; it's still exaggerated. You do not want to eat a little and often? No problem, eat just as you usually would one or two fasting twenty-four hours a week.

14. To win in confidence. If you lose weight, dress better and buy new ones, you

cannot feel more confident. It's a great feeling!

CHAPTER FOUR
Intermittent Fasting/Burn Fat

Women are more prone to have excess fat than men. The main reason is reproduction. The woman's body is continuously preparing to feed her baby. But how much fat is that?

One way to determine the amount of fat a person carries is to use BMI (Body Mass Index). It is an estimate that gives a rating to a person's height and weight.

For years, we've been told that the big is beautiful and the truth is that beauty is in the eyes of the beholder, but we cannot keep saying it. Overweight is not attractive and is not healthy. The number of Western women who are overweight to the extent that they pose a risk to their health exceeds 50%. Some health conditions caused by the transport of excess fat include:

- Heart failure: An increase in heart size caused by thickening of the heart muscle means that the heart cannot pump enough blood to other organs in the body.
- Menstrual disorders cause severe pain and bleeding or missed rules.
- Fat accumulation around the liver can cause inflammation and possibly cirrhosis.
- Stones irritate when the bile hardens into stone-like pieces.
- Diabetes: which is the body's inability to maintain healthy blood sugar.

This number is higher than in previous generations, so what is the cause?

Overweight children are more likely to have excess fat in adulthood. Our fast-paced lifestyle has led us to eat a lot of food waste, and the wrong choice of food can become a habit that makes our body crave for eating the wrong foods and is an essential factor. Our lives are sedentary. Many children now spend too much time watching television, playing a computer or playing video games instead of playing outside.

If a child eats bad foods and does not exercise enough, his body stores fats instead of burning them. If we allow our children to develop bad habits, it becomes a way of life. Statistics show that the thicker a child is, the less confidence he has in him. These character traits reach adulthood and can prevent a woman from being motivated to act. She thinks life will always be like that.

The negative messages sent to our brain as we grow up are compelling. We must change our mind before we can take the first step. Your brain controls the release of hormones to burn fat after each meal. When we eat, we need a diet that guides our hormones so that we may lose fat.

From time to time, fasting has become a popular way of using the body's natural ability to burn fat, to lose fat in a shorter time. However, many people want to know if it works with an occasional fast and how exactly it works. When you spend a long time without eating, your body changes the way it creates hormones and enzymes, which can be an advantage for fat loss. These are the main benefits of fasting and its benefits.

Hormones are the basis of metabolic functions, including the rate of fat burning. Growth hormone produces your body and stimulates the breakdown of fat in the body to give it energy. When you starve for a moment, your body starts to increase growth hormone production. Also, fasting helps reduce the amount of insulin in the blood, ensuring that your body burns fat instead of storing it.

Short-term fasting for 12 to 72 hours increases metabolism and adrenaline levels, forcing you to burn more calories. Also, fasting people get more energy with increased adrenaline, which helps them not to feel tired, although they usually do not receive calories. Although you may think that fasting should reduce heat, the body compensates for it by providing a way to burn calories.

Most people who eat every 3 to 5 hours burn mostly sugar rather than fat. Prolonged fasting activates your metabolism to burn fat. At the end of the 24-hour fasting day, your body consumed glycogen stores in the early hours and wasted about 18 hours of body fat. For people who are regularly active but still struggle with fat loss, intermittent fasting can help increase fat loss without the need for more exercise or drastically changing the diet.

Another advantage of occasional fasting is that it permanently restores the body. It lasts a day or two and, without eating, it changes a person's desire, which makes them less hungry with time. If you have problems with a constant hunger for food, intermittent fasting can help your body adapt to periods of food inactivity and not to feel hungry always. Many people notice that they are starting to eat healthier and better-controlled foods when they eat one day a week.

Occasional hunger is different, but it is usually recommended about a day a week. During the day, a person can have a liquid smoothie, nutritious or other low-calorie option. As the body adapts to intermittent fasting, this is usually not necessary. Intermittent fasting helps reduce body fat stores by altering metabolism by breaking down fat instead of sugar or muscle. Many people have used it effectively, and it is an easy way to make a useful change. For people struggling with stubborn and tired fats from the traditional diet, occasional fasting is a simple and effective option for fat loss and a healthier lifestyle.

Most people want to lose weight to look better. Many people want to get rid of their damaged muscles and abs, but very few do because they do not do what it takes to reach that low body fat percentage. If you want to be broken, weightlifting is only part of the equation. The second part is to eliminate body fat, and I want to show you how you can do it in a short time.

I recently started a program of weight loss and muscle development that includes occasional fasting. If you do not know, this is a strategy that does not eat long. At first, I was skeptical because I always heard terrible things about skipping meals. In the world of health, it is common knowledge that not eating food often slows down your metabolism and sends your body into a state of starvation that will store more fat. What I found is not valid. The opposite is closer to the truth. Eating regularly every day will put your body in "fat storage" mode because you think you are preparing for hunger or drought. If you do not eat for a long time, the body goes into fat-burning mode and also allows rapid detoxification of the body, which has many benefits.

From time to time, fasting can be done in different ways. The method that I found most useful is a daily publication from 16h to 20h. It means within 4 to 8 hours. This often involves skipping breakfast and lunch. Since then, I have seen a dramatic increase in energy levels, especially in the morning, as well as a drop in blood pressure and a dramatic decrease in body fat percentage. During intermittent fasting for four months, I lost 15 pounds and gained a lot of muscle at the same time. I finally had the torn look that I always wanted.

On the no chance that you need to get thinner, consume fat, develop your muscles or all the above, the occasional fast is probably one of the best things you can do for yourself.

Burn fat quickly and easily:

Some weight loss tips do not work at all, but others work miracles, and I think I've found one. I have been experimenting with weight loss for four months, and this has allowed me to develop my muscles while losing 15 pounds. Many do not know this method, but it has the potential to transform their body completely. Then I want to tell you what I know.

Four months ago, I started doing occasional publications. Fasting, if you have never heard of it, is when you do not eat solid foods. We all fast while we sleep, but the reason we never enjoy it is that we do not do it fast enough. Most people drink as soon as they wake up and just before going to bed. This is bad for several reasons. Since it continually feeds your body, you must always feed your digestive system with blood, leaving little to stay prone to other parts of the body, such as your brain. If you can increase the time you are hungry, your body will have more time to clean and repair. This is essential for good health. Fasting has proven to be one of the best ways to reduce blood pressure, cholesterol and blood sugar. It is also ideal for improving mood, increasing energy and burning fat fast. These are just a few of the many benefits that fasting can sometimes offer, but they should be enough to attract you to try this method yourself.

From time to time, fasting is very easy; as long as you get used to skipping a meal or two a day. Do not worry, it means you can eat more when it's time to eat. Sometimes fasting does not require you to count calories, change the foods you eat or even participate in an exercise routine. All the benefits of fasting come directly from the time you spend eating. The more time you can eat without eating, the more you will benefit from it. If you can reduce the time you spend eating daily, you will experience a considerable number of benefits. The

Intermittent Fasting for Women

normal way to do this is to skip breakfast, as this will increase the time you spend quickly. For faster results, skip breakfast and lunch and eat all your food inside the window for 4 to 8 hours. If you can pay at least 16 hours of fasting each day, you will experience significant weight loss and many other health benefits.

> You Lose Fat by Fasting from Time to Time:

As a skinny and fat guy, you have probably tried to lose weight with limited success. I tried a lot of diets. I started eating high protein foods 6 to 8 times a day, and I lost fat to get it back because I was tired of eating small, healthy snacks. After a year and a half of training, I discovered the benefits of a casual job by reading Eat Stop Eat. To this day, Eat Stop Eat is my favourite nutrition book. In an occasional post, divide the day into two phases:

Phase 1: 8 hours of feeding.

Phase 2: fasting phase of 16 hours.

By doing this, you will not be able to eat more than 2 or 3 solid meals a day, and the fasting phase of 16 hours will allow you to lose fat. This is a practical approach for a lean and fat man because to lose fat, and you must consume fewer calories more than you burn. In my opinion, the most enjoyable and fun way to lose fat is to practice casual fasting in your lifestyle because it is straightforward. An added benefit is that many find that they are very productive during the fasting phase as they do not spend their mornings preparing breakfast and eating.

If you are a student like me, the casual job might look like this:

07:00: Wake up and have a cup of coffee.

12:00 - 08:00: power phase.

08:00 - 12:00: After the phase.

As you can see above, it's simple: instead of having breakfast, drink a good cup of coffee (no sugar) and stay productive until noon to avoid eating. When your 8-hour feeding phase begins, you eat 2 or 3 solid meals that feed your workout. After your last lunch, you can relax and enjoy the night until you go to bed. I have had success with this approach, even though I eat what I want at each meal, as long as most of my consumption is healthy.

Therefore, if you apply the occasional fast in your lifestyle, you can forget everything:

- Eat small, unsatisfactory meals every 2-3 hours.

- Get up early for breakfast.

- Experiment with an insulin tip in the afternoon.

- the number of calories.

Also, I go out and skip the fasting phase once a week, but that did not stop me from losing weight.

That said, many ask: what can I consume during the fasting phase? The answer is coffee, tea and sugar-free gum. The most essential thing is to stay hydrated during the fasting phase to avoid hunger.

In short, here are the benefits of occasional display:

- Easy to implement.

- Eat satisfying meals.

- You lose fat, and you gain muscle.

- Skip breakfast and sleep.

> **How to Lose Belly Fat for Women?**

Women are prone to weight gain more than men, especially in the tummy region of the body. All the ladies are in a bid to achieve a flat stomach because that is supposed to be a sign of a well-shaped physique. Though it is achievable, attaining a flat tummy is a task that needs serious work and effort. Instructions to lose tummy fat for women is a multidimensional inquiry with numerous responses to it. One needs to adopt an energy strategy to lose midsection fat. One has to take a systematic approach to lose belly fat. There are many ways like dieting, exercising, boosting one's metabolism, etc.

One of the ways how to lose belly fat for women is eating frequent meals. This helps boost the metabolic rate of the body. Getting five to six meals a day will save women from overeating or binging over junk food.

High metabolic rate burns food at a faster rate which prevents the accumulation of fat near the tummy region. Nutrition is essential while losing weight, be it in any part of the body. Eating right is of prime importance. Women should keep track of the intake of calories every day and sometimes also consume more calories for instant belly fat loss. They should include whole grains, fruits, skimmed milk, brown rice, lean meat, vegetables and additionally at least six grams of fish oil in their diet. They should also not skip breakfast to remain on the lighter side of the weighing scale.

Also, another way for women to lose belly fat is the rigorous exercise of exercising. Women need to follow an intense program of both cardio and weight training in their routine. That is an effective way of how to lose belly fat for women. Doing cardio continuously for long sessions leads to cortisol accumulation which leads to belly fat. Hence women should intersperse cardio with weight training in their exercise regime to achieve those washboard abs or the flat stomach that they desire.

Consuming a lot of fluids can also help reduce fat. Women should drink water so much so that they always remain hydrated, and water will help burn all the excess fat. How to lose fat for women is more comfortable if they consume green tea regularly. Green tea dilutes all the fatty solids, and therefore, women get the desired flat stomach.

Eating a lot of fibre food like fruits and vegetables also helps reduce weight in women. Some of the hormonal changes that take place in a woman's body are also responsible for belly fat. High levels of progesterone in their body right before menstruation gives rise to a fat belly during the menstruating week, which is a difficult aspect for most women. Fibres help women to feel fuller and healthier, also cutting off craving pangs. The MUFA's in fibre foods also helps reduce cholesterol levels along with diminishing belly fat. Women should take at least 35 grams of fibre in their diet. Hence the answer to how to lose weight for women is sufficiently answered in the above steps.

➢ **Techniques that You Can Use to Get a Sexy Flat Stomach:**

1) The diet does not affect abdominal fat loss or general fat loss. They indeed work in the short term, but in the long run, you get all the weight and more. Diet slows down your metabolism. What you need is an appropriate diet program that works with and not against your body.

2) Abdominal exercises are not practical traditional abdominal exercises, such as the stomach or abdominal machines, are the least effective method for eliminating abdominal fat. Instead, make hammocks to train your abdominal muscles.

3) Long and slow cardio is not going to help. Almost all the women in the gym do long and slow cardiovascular exercises, and most of them look the same as they did a few months ago. Some of the thinnest people never make any weak or traditional cardio. Try a high-intensity interval training instead. HIIT training minutes are high-intensity exercises followed by low-intensity exercise minutes. HIIT training burns fat much faster than traditional cardio.

4) Do body-building exercises to be or stay very lean, and you will have to do weight training exercises. It does not matter whether you like it or not, and the important thing is that it works to lose weight fast. Do not worry, and you'll look like a bodybuilder. It will not happen. Cardio burns fat during training, but body-building burns fats after exercise, but sugar during exercise.

5) Eat more often. Most women only eat two or three times a day and often have a snack or fruit. If you want to burn stubborn belly fat quickly, you should eat at least five or recommended six per 24 hours. Then your body signals your metabolism "hello, reactivate yourself".

> ➢ How to Lose Fat Around Your Hips?

➢ **Exercise at Home - hula hoping:**
It's a problem. It has been proven that the hula hoop offers an excellent tonic, firming and complete definition at the waist and hip. That's why he goes crazy all over the country. What you can do is buy a heavy hoop. They are more expensive than a circle, $ 15-20, but they are worth it.

If you do not get a heavy hoop, do not even bother to make one, because it will fall more easily on the floor before you also have the opportunity to twist your waist twice. The extra weight slows the hoops to the point where the hips will have no trouble balancing their balance.

Ten minutes of hula-hello will make your hips thrive in the world of good.

➢ **Nutritional Advice- Add protein shakes as snacks:**

Most people make the mistake of using protein shakes as meal replacements. This is not good because they usually do not provide enough calories, so you want to eat before your next meal. The solution is to eat healthy foods and use protein shakes as snacks or mini-meals. The added protein helps you to speed up your metabolism while controlling your blood sugar.

➢ Burn Fat Legs by Counting Calories:

On the one hand, the Atkins diet seems logical to say that carbohydrates can gain fat if they eat it in excess. However, this is not a reason to exclude them entirely from your diet. If you get rid of it completely, you will not like the results.

Because carbohydrates are a vital source of energy, their elimination will inevitably make you feel sick and tired. It is better to continue to eat but in moderation.

Well, every person has the number of calories required to be consumed each day. For example, an average woman needs about 2,000 calories to reach her "maintenance level". The reason many people are overweight is pure because they consume more energy than necessary.

Let's say that a woman eats 2,250 calories a day while she has only 2,000. This, of course, exceeds her maintenance level, which means there is extra energy that her body will not use. So what about this energy? You have it, and it gets bigger.

This is what seems to me so essential, and that simplifies the idea of weight loss. Let's say that this woman only eats 1,500 calories a day for several weeks. Of course, as the body does not pull all the energy it needs from food, it will go into energy stores and burn mainly that excess fat. This means that you can quickly start losing fat from your thigh without having to think about a stylish diet.

On the other hand, it is very complicated to count the calories of everything you eat, but it can be easy to make a change. One idea is to reduce the number of portions during a meal. You see, although some people eat healthy enough and never eat snacks, they can still be overweight because of the size of their meals, which equates too much higher energy levels than necessary.

However, if you have the motivation to burn this fat, the process of checking the caloric content of your food is not a considerable time constraint and must become second nature. With this low-calorie mind-set, it will only take a few weeks before you notice a noticeable difference in size. So take control of the size of your portions today and enjoy the fastest way to lose weight.

> **Activities You Can Do Every Day:**

Consuming fat and disposing of those additional calories is a test for the majority of us. We often think about how far the gym is, and sometimes we do not have a lot of time to go to the gym after work. If you are starting a weight loss program or want to take small steps to change your lifestyle, you can do it alone and outside the gym.

First, the best way to lose weight and burn fat is to change your lifestyle and habits. When you have begun, you will never feel constrained to endeavour to get in shape.

You will find below simple and natural fat loss exercises. These exercises are things you can do each day and whenever during the day. In the event that you put shortly every day playing and picking these exercises as opposed to sitting on the lounge chair before a TV show or perusing a book, you can certainly see the benefits of these useful but straightforward activities.

1. Walk. Walking is one of the most natural exercises and again, a great way to lose weight. On the weekends, you can choose to walk the dog, walk in the park, walk in the block, walk in the morning or just walk.

Walking does not only burn these fats, but its benefits are infinite.

2. Jog. Jogging is also an excellent cardiovascular exercise to burn fat, especially around the abdomen.

3. Take the stairs instead of the elevator.

4. Walk around the office. Spend a few minutes of walking in your office.

5. Cycling. Just like walking or running, cycling is also a great cardiovascular exercise.

6. Do the housework. If you do not want to go to the gym but want to keep your body moving, clean it up. Wash the dishes, clean the windows of everything away from the sofa and the bed.

7. Garden or mow the lawn. By using your green thumb, you lose that fat.

8. Play sports. If you want a fun and exciting cardiovascular exercise, you can practice a sport or learn a new one. Swimming, tennis, skiing and other ball games can all be functional cardiovascular exercises to lose

fat and improve health. They are also much more fun than other forms of activities.

9. Do yoga. This conditions not only your body but also your mind.

10. Try to dance. Dance, belly dancing or any modern dance can also burn fat.

11. Join aerobics classes. You can do it at the gym or home with an aerobics CD.

12. Do the abs. If you like to burn belly fat and abdominal tone, you can do sit-ups after cardiovascular exercise.

> ## Seven Exercise Tips for Losing Weight Fast:

No woman on this planet does not dream of a slim figure. But the reality is that most of us cannot lose weight or lose fat because of our unhealthy foods and lifestyles, reduced physical activity or not, our strenuous work schedules, our stress, our anxiety and so little time. Let's stop blaming all these external factors and see how easy and fast it is to lose fat.

❖ Look at the clock to lose weight: It is essential to consider the time of your snack or meal before your workout. Something new may seem to you, and the first thing that comes to mind is how it will help you lose fat. Of course, it will. It gives you extra strength for longer and harder workouts, which can help you burn more calories and lose fat. But remember that the time is crucial i.e., eating closer to an exercise program increases blood supply to the stomach and harms its performance.

❖ Breathe properly to lose weight: The right way to inhale through the nose and not through the mouth. Breathing through the nose helps to stabilize the heart rate and increase endurance and, as a result, enables you to lose fat. It works very similar to a pre-workout snack for fat loss. Increasing endurance can help you exercise more and burn more calories, which will be the best way to lose fat. Do not pay attention if you do not feel natural. You will soon get used to the practice.

- ❖ Keep the cardio for the end: When you exercise to lose weight and gain weight, do some form of cardiovascular exercise first. This is because the body takes about fifteen minutes to warm up; only after that, it starts to burn fat. Therefore, to lose weight properly, it is advisable to warm up your body thoroughly with weight exercises before cycling or other cardiovascular exercises.

- ❖ Diversity is the spice of life: It's another useful tip for fast and effective weight loss. Do not give in to the same form of exercise day after day. The body gets bored quickly, and you end up burning fewer calories during the day. This breaks the whole program to lose fat. Every day, you should perform different exercises. It's refreshing for the mind and the body.

- ❖ Do not lose weight: Cracking or drooling is terrible because it inhibits the amount of oxygen entering the body. So stop going down on the wheel of your exercise bike as it can take a long time to lose weight and fat effectively.

❖ Periodicity of exercises: Although the best way to lose weight and exercise with fat is as intense and slow as possible, it is not recommended to do so if you are starting an exercise program. It is best to train at regular intervals to lose weight quickly. This will not only increase your stamina but will also help you lose weight faster.

❖ Lightweight exercises to lose fat: Do exercises that can improve muscle tone as it is a safe way to burn more calories.

Regular application of these main training tips can help you lose a lot of weight and lose more and more weight. The dark figure you want will not look so far.

➢ Abdominal Fat:

Abdominal fat is the most common problem in the body. The fat usually accumulates in the abdominal area, giving a bulging belly that looks uncomfortable. Exercises on how to lose those bumps in your stomach are a way to lubricate fats. Abdominal or abdominal exercises are the most common form of exercise used to reduce height. The three main exercises for the abdomen designed to pull the waist are:

➢ **Abs Against the Ball:**

Running an abs ball proved to be more effective compared to a healthy belly on the ground. This requires a balance, which makes it difficult to maintain stability. The balloon helps you specifically target your abdominal muscles by isolating your abdominal muscles, creating more resistance and helping to contract your abdominal muscles.

➢ **Leg Lifts in a Supine Position:**

This targets the lower abdomen muscles. Eliminate the belly that is to blame for the bulging tummy. They are designed to burn fat effectively to appear soberer, without lumps. Perfect for beach lovers, you can now wear a thinner belly.

> **Lateral Cracks in the Ball:**

The idea is technically the same as that of the stomach, but the goal is to eliminate the love handles by slamming them. Making a belly on the ball will help you burn your hands in the stomach and reduce these love handles. The lateral muscles are responsible for creating a curved look for you to look better.

These exercises target all the major muscles in your abdomen to help you burn the superficial fat in your abdominal cavity. The effectiveness of these exercises depends on the intensity, so the harder it is, the better the results. So think of challenging your body and increasing your playoffs and your reps.

> Exercise Burns Fat:

It is not enough to do a low abdominal workout. You must also understand the basics of this training. For example, know that this exercise is not a promising technique for losing abdominal fat. Every exercise you do to lose abdominal fat helps you lose fat throughout your body, not to lose fat only from a proper part of your body. But the good news is that it will strengthen the muscle core and tone when performing lower abdominal exercises.

To lose fat, you must combine strength training and healthy eating. Do not worry if you do not want to develop muscle tone because you will not do it. As you move towards a healthier lifestyle, you will experience weight loss and get a well-adjusted body. After that, you can start doing low-abdominal exercises.

Below are some of the most effective exercises for lower abdominal exercises to get you started:

➢ **Walk Alternately with Elongated Legs:** Start rest on your back with your hands under your buttocks. Lift your legs. Make a contraction of the abscess. You know that you are doing the right thing if you feel tense in your environment.

Lower your right leg slowly, less than 5 inches off the ground. Wait for a second, lift your right leg again and lower your left leg slightly as you would with your right hand. Lift your left leg back. Repeat this step a dozen times. Increase the repetition as you go.

➢ Lift the Legs:

This exercise is similar to the first. Same starting position i.e., lie on your back, hands under the buttocks. The legs must also be straight. Lower the abdomen while slowly lowering the legs. But not too little for the foot to touch the ground. Feet should be a few inches from the ground. Maintain an abdominal contraction by doing this. Repeat this exercise a dozen times and slowly increase the repetition as you progress.

➢ Reverse Lapels:

Lie on your back with your both hands under your buttocks. Lift your legs as if you had done it in the two previous exercises. Now, bend your knees at a 90-degree angle. Keep this flexibility while contracting the abs. Maintain the tension.

Spread your knees slowly and lower your legs straight. Stop when your feet touch the ground. Stay in this position and slowly bend both your knees again. Now your knees should touch your torso. Tighten your stomach firmly while doing this. Repeat this minor exercise about five times. Increase the repetition as you go.

> ➢ **The Following Includes the Main Fat Loss Exercises:**

Boxing:

Boxing is a remarkable sport that burns about 613 calories per hour. In addition to this, boxing is the best exercise for burning fat and allows you to learn some useful self-defence techniques while burning fat. Plus, you would be incredibly flexible in handling the bag, boxing, fighting and speed that's part of the sport.

Burpees:

Burpees burn 546 calories per hour and are new weight control exercises. Also, they provide all the muscles in your body with an effective workout that builds muscle mass and increases the amount of body fat, you burn each day.

Jump Rope:

Threading a rope requires resistance, but it's a great exercise that you can do anytime, anywhere. Burn about 798 calories per hour and requires no equipment, just a skipping rope and you're ready to start.

Jump Squats:

Squat-jumping is the best exercise for fat loss. It is a simple but effective weight movement that exercises all the leg muscles and burns an average of 900 calories per hour.

Climbing is a great fun, challenging and unique exercise. Climbing alone burns 749 calories per hour, but it also gives all the muscles in your body an intense workout that increases your muscle mass and has a long-term positive effect on the amount of body fat, you burn.

Running:

Running is another best fat loss exercise that allows you to burn a lot of fat, but also requires endurance options that you can develop through constant practice. Also, this will enable you to enjoy the outdoors while increasing your vitamin D level. Running burns about 920 calories per hour.

Indoor Cycling:

Indoor cycling is the best exercise that involves pedalling with music at different intensities. It is an excellent fat burner that burns about 700 calories per hour and also works very well to strengthen the muscles of the lower body.

Step-ups:

The procedures are a simple cardiovascular exercise that works well by targeting the muscles of the lower body and can be performed in a narrow and compact space. The improvements increase by 972 calories per hour.

Cardio:

If you want to burn more fat with cardio, you need to make sure that you are doing intense exercises that stimulate many muscle groups. I hate elliptical and stationary bikes because they are not fierce and only tend the muscles.

The best cardiovascular exercises for fat loss are running, rowing, jumping rope, swimming, kickboxing, etc. Each of these exercises exhausts many muscle groups. You often receive them as strength training and cardio.

Bodybuilding:

Developing muscle tissue is very important if you want to lose fat. The muscles increase your metabolism, which not only allows you to burn calories while exercising but also throughout the day. This is a double advantage.

Fat burning exercises are those that work in more than one muscle group. These include squats, lunges, chest slits, pumps, chin, underline, need for pushing, etc. Contrary to what one might think, sitting is not an excellent exercise for burning fat.

> ➢ How Often do I Have to Exercise to Lose Fat?

Exercise is also essential, and brisk walking is not as effective at burning calories as an intense workout or an intense aerobics session. Therefore, the question of how often you have to exercise to lose fat cannot be solved. However, if you acquire the qualifications above, you can answer, and it is "as often as you like".

It also depends on how much fat you want to lose. If you feel that your metabolism and your weight are in balance, when you do not increase, or you lose weight, then the more you exercise, the faster you will lose weight. This weight loss should be oily if most exercises are aerobic (which includes oxygen), although any initial rapid weight loss is probably an excess of water.

There are two types of exercises: aerobic exercises that involve a lot of breathing (running, swimming, cycling, rowing, levelling, etc.) and anaerobic exercises, which means little or no breathing (weightlifting, speed races), the cells in your body use glucose and oxygen to generate energy. Once your blood glucose is diluted, and the carbohydrates in your diet become glucose, your body fat is converted into a carbohydrate source that metabolises more glucose to provide the energy you need to continue exercising.

In the less practical anaerobic exercises, there is not enough oxygen to convert glucose into energy. Your body will, therefore, use known alternative mechanisms such as lactic acid fermentation and anaerobic glycolysis to produce energy. It is not as effective as aerobic glycolysis so that anaerobic activity will result in less weight loss, but more muscle fibre formation. Then train and "exercise" and discuss "how much" you need to be more specific in what you have in mind.

However, to lose fat, you must burn more calories than you consume. The answer to this question, therefore, depends in part on your diet. The fewer carbs you eat including fats, grains, starch and sugars, the less exercise you need to lose fat. However, there is also a fact that the more muscle you have, the higher the metabolic rate at which you consume more calories during your sleep or rest. Again, you can exercise less than usual to lose weight.

There are ways to determine the number of calories you burn during a typical day. If you know your body fat index (BFI), what is

Intermittent Fasting for Women

the fat content, you can calculate a relatively fast basic metabolic rate. Otherwise, it depends on your age, weight and size. However, most people have no idea of their BFI, so they rely heavily on educated guesses that figures calculate the number of exercises needed to lose weight at a reasonable rate (about 2 to 3 pounds per week).

What many do is adopt a specific workout regimen and then record their daily and weekly weight loss. They will usually lose a few pounds quickly as they remove the excess water in their cells and then reduce the rate of weight loss as they burn fat contained in their fat cells to use as energy. From this, they can judge the amount of extra exercise they need to achieve a specific fat loss rate.

Fat is not just disappearing: the body has used it as a source of carbohydrate to convert it to glucose after consuming the carbohydrate content of your diet. If you replace the sugar in the diet with protein, you will lose fat more quickly because your body will depend on the carbohydrate component of the protein for your glucose and then switch to fat. The amino acid content of the protein will be used to develop more muscle fibres, which will increase your metabolic rate, that will result in a higher conversion of fats to glucose.

Therefore, maintaining the right amount of protein in your diet instead of regular carbohydrates can speed up fat loss and muscle growth. However, keep in mind the need for a low-fat diet that allows you to get enough fat-soluble vitamins A, E and K so you do not just eat protein. That's one of the weaknesses of Atkins' protein-rich diet: the need for extra nutritional supplements, and that's where Atkins made a lot of money.

CHAPTER FIVE

The Easiest Way to Improve Your Life

Fasting provides the essential benefits of weight loss, which is excellent, but also an internal sense of accomplishment and control of our body and weight. Much of our life is beyond our power to think about how good it will be to control this region. It works very well for your self-esteem; You are proud to lose weight and control your body. It's not about fasting for political reasons or drawing attention to a specific cause, and this publication is for you and allows you to reach your weight loss goals.

Now the question is, how to fast? I am a big fan of what is called "fasting", which is a practice, a speed at a time. It's flexible. You fast 1 to 2 days a week, the days you want. So, if you have an event or projects, you do not have to reject or attend, but postpone it to another day quickly. This type of fasting also allows people to maintain a moderate to a rigorous exercise routine if they wish.

Starting slowly and getting used to the lifestyle is the best way to begin your publication program. This will give you a lot more success. Plans at a moderate pace sometimes lose their appeal because people become discouraged and lose interest. Start slowly to ensure success!

It's a good idea to consult a publication like this one to improve not only your diet and your fitness, but also for many additional benefits of fasting, including the sense of discipline, better well-being, A real opportunity to rejuvenate your body and an antidote to starvation. The lives we all live.

> Nutritional Supplements Can Help You Every Day of Your Life:

Nutritional supplements can provide you with these nutrients, and a wise purchase can be very beneficial. However, it is crucial to understand that you need to consider more than the cost of the supplement to get the best value for your nutritional budget. Therefore, changing your diet and using dietary supplements for diabetes can help promote better metabolism and overcome abnormalities. Anyone interested in a healthy lifestyle, not just diabetics, should explore the various vitamins and minerals recommended to supplement the average American diet. These investigations suggest that the biochemical lopsided characteristics that healthful enhancements can address themselves are quick reasons for dependence.

It is best to slowly add dietary supplements to your diet, starting with small doses and gradually increasing the amounts recommended by the manufacturers. It is also best to take certain supplements, such as herbal remedies that can stimulate the body's processes, which sometimes allows the body to rest occasionally without supplements. Home-grown drugs and dietary enhancements are not controlled by the Food and Drug Administration (FDA) as prescription drugs, unlike over-the-counter medications. In 2004, the World Health Organization (WHO) published guidelines on the use of medicinal plants, including recommendations on cultivation, collection, classification, quality control, storage, labelling and distribution. The formulation has results: bodybuilding supplements help you gain weight. Sports supplements should help athletes keep playing until the last second.

Nutritional supplements can take different shapes and sizes. Many dietary supplements can make a big difference in your life. Nutritional supplements are exactly what they mean. The body needs nutrients, minerals and different supplements to remain stable. If handled with care, natural supplements can be an integral part of your arthritis treatment plan. But the keyword is careful.

As should be obvious, wholesome enhancements can assist you with getting thinner and improve your wellbeing. Remember that we recommend supplements that help your body, not supplements, diet pills, etc. Nutritional supplements can cause such a change in middle-aged women. At higher doses than usual, dietary supplements may have a positive pharmacological effect. In any chronic disease, oxidative stress increases and leads to an accumulation of problems.

If surgery is planned or an adverse event occurs, the physician should ask the patient for any alternative medication. This will allow the patient and the physician to discuss possible adverse interactions and plan for a potential interruption of the

Intermittent Fasting for Women

program before surgery. Ask the help of grocery store employees or health professionals to find reliable brands. Contact the supplement company directly and ask questions about quality control and the Radical Oxygen Absorption Test (ORAC). Nutrient B6 is fundamental for the creation of serotonin and keeps the resistant framework stable.

Natural products are essential because they facilitate and accelerate the healing process. Our products are under no circumstances treated or treated.

It depends on whom you ask. As per the FDA, the sexual impacts of aphrodisiacs depend on old stories and not on certainties. For instance, it might be alluring to control severe tasting fixings to cover their desire (for example, a container or tablet) instead of incorporating them into the nutritional composition (e.g., powdered or tacky). Accordingly, the invention also provides a pharmaceutical package or kit containing one or more containers filled with one or more ingredients of the nutritional composition of the device (for example, a

Intermittent Fasting for Women

nourishment supplement as powders and cases containing tea green and caffeine).

My biggest objection to props is that people see them as an easy way out; They consider meal replacements or protein shakes as a complete meal. Drinks, bars, cookies, whatever, were supposed to "supplement" what whole foods cannot give you, and therefore the importance of combining carbohydrates and proteins.

Supplements strengthen cartilage and joints, allowing for greater flexibility, bone strength and pain relief. Natural supplements have become a popular alternative treatment for arthritis and osteoporosis. Taking a handful of vitamins is not helpful and is not "natural". There are vitamins and minerals that, at an extra dose, may be useful in certain situations. You should discuss this with your doctor. The encouraged course of action is to take a particular formula for several months.

Nutritional supplements can provide these nutrients and with a careful purchase, can be very beneficial. However, it is essential to understand that you need to consider more than the cost of the supplement to get the best value for your nutritional budget. Therefore, changing your diet and using dietary supplements for diabetes can help promote better metabolism and overcome abnormalities. Anyone interested in a healthy lifestyle, not just diabetics, should explore the various vitamins and minerals recommended to complement the average American diet. These studies suggest that the biochemical instability, that nutritional excess can correct, are themselves direct causes of addiction.

The hardest part is to devote yourself to a healthy diet to give your body the nutrition it needs to age and stay active. Another aspect is the apparent need for people with diabetes to consume nutritious drinks with flavoured drinks that help maintain blood sugar and do not add excess calories but have sufficient nutritional value and attractive taste.

➢ Increase your Confidence with Weight Loss:

Lack of trust is common in many people around the world for several reasons. In my opinion, overweight and poor health seems to play an essential role in how you feel about yourself. If you are not satisfied with your appearance, you will never reach your potential, because uncertainty will forbid you from achieving what you want to make. If you're going to succeed in life, do not just aim more, but do more. Be healthy and fit, and you will feel incredible & natural to accomplish more. If you have trouble losing weight, you probably have difficulties in other areas of your life. Losing weight cannot only improve your health and confidence but also your success in almost everything you do.

If you have trouble losing weight, I want to tell you that there is hope for you because once I was in your place. I have spent years trying to lose my ideal weight and have never been able to achieve the desired results. But recently, I started doing things that significantly improved my health and worked wonders with my weight loss. I want to exchange with you some of these things.

First, I started the transition to a healthier diet. This is the key if you want to lose weight without getting it back. However, do not overeat. Otherwise, you will struggle to maintain a healthy diet. Start by gradually incorporating more fruits and vegetables into your diet and start progressively eliminating all the sweet and processed foods. A normal way to do this is to start buying healthy foods when you go to the store and altogether avoid rays with processed foods. Avoid as much as possible foods in boxes or cans. It's a slow process. Do not try to do it overnight, but recognise that eating healthy is a way of life, not a diet.

The second method I use to lose weight fast is called intermittent fasting. This involves skipping one or two meals a day to give body the time needed to detoxify and burn fat. Intermittent fasting has several advantages. I recommend you to learn more and include it in your routine.

> **Control your Energy, do not Let It Control You:**

As a small child, energy flows continuously. Some children are "treated" for abundant energy. However, as we get older, our power seems to be diminishing, and we want to have the strength we had as children. Unfortunately, stress, fatigue, poor nutrition, lack of sleep, extra work, emotional barriers and many other sources reduce energy levels. What we do not realize is that we control our energy levels. Lack of energy is a self-inflicted disease (if desired). We must return to the basic principles of life as we were when we were children and revive our source of youth energy steadily.

Think about it when you were a child, you made fun of the world, you loved life and absorbed all the information you could. You lived life moment by moment. You probably ate a better-balanced meal than you have now, went to bed early, had lunch, smiled, laughed, hoped to dream, was active, looked fresh whenever you could, and ate only sweet food on birthdays. Think of all the things you love, that you were passionate about and that you had lived as a child. Is it the majority of them, and the ones you could start integrating into your life today?

I will help you to follow the right path. On the one hand, remove all unnecessary sugars from your diet. Sugar is a medicine in the body. Our body has not been designed to absorb processed and refined foods stored with sugars and carbohydrates. Do you recall what your mother always told you? Eat this green bean! Eat healthy, unprocessed and natural foods as much as possible. Foods produced on land or wood, foods of animal origin and animal fats are what the body is designed to eat. When the body receives nutrients, it can decompose and act more efficiently. Pay attention to food labels because sugar can appear on anything (tomato sauce, vinaigrette, biscuits). Eliminating sugar will boost your system and, as a result, increase energy levels, restore hungry cells and naturally balance your body's systems. Fat loss could even be an added benefit.

Because of more energy when your diet changes, you will feel more active. Activity is a natural stimulant for the body when performed in specific settings exercise for power use for 20 to 30 minutes a day, including weight training and cardio training. Exercising more than 45 minutes a day will cause a decrease in energy as the body will begin to draw power from its protein stores (in other words, muscles) Naturally after exercise. Concentrate on improving the strength of your body through bodybuilding. Performing several sets of push-ups, and squats can be difficult enough to get you started. No gym membership required. Concentrate on improving the natural function of your body before adopting more demanding exercise plans. As with any exercise program, spend one day a week without exercise to allow your body to recover up to 100% of its energy level.

The quality of food is not only a crucial factor in energy production but also a question of time. Do you remember that after a long day playing outside, your mother would be ready for dinner or at least a healthy snack? What he did not realize that he was contributing to his energy level, exhausted by the activity of the day to restore his body immediately. Try to eat your biggest meal of the day after an event or exercise. Eating less than an hour after exercise is essential to regain your body and energy the next day. The muscles break down during intense muscle training or cardiovascular exercises (hence muscle pain). To restore these muscles more effectively, food is essential for these cells to start repairing themselves. This not only assists in speeding up the recovery process but also to prevent pain in the coming days.

Another critical factor that I mentioned in the introductory paragraph is the dream. The body is better revitalized for 7 to 8 hours of sleep (for most people). It is recommended to sleep before 10PM. because the body sleeps harder between eleven o'clock in the evening and two in the morning. Make the most of your sleep schedule before 10:00 AM. or 10:30 PM. Another reason to get enough sleep is to fill the brain and the body. When a person is tired, the body needs carbohydrates (in other words: sugar), While it is the ultimate source of energy that it needs, resulting in a sudden increase in insulin which exacerbates the problem. So go to bed at 10 PM, and all the rest will go smoothly.

The last element to increase energy is exercise with intermittent fasting. As a youth, we tend to think that we should eat at 8 AM in the morning because it's breakfast time, and if we are hungry or not, we should eat at noon because lunch is always served at this time and we must go back, Eat at 5 PM. For the same common reason, it's excellent and unpleasant, but most of us rest where we eat coffee and a snack, whether we are hungry or not. Some people have a meal for the night before going to bed, which is a big no-no, as it interferes with our quiet sleep time of 10 hours. At 2:00 Pithed body will try to break down the abundance of sugar we consume before closing our eyes during the night, which will not allow our system to rest completely. Let's go back to fasting, although sometimes when we eat or consume abundant glycaemic foods, the body takes longer to digest. Also, a meal high in sugar may cause other symptoms such as bloating, nausea, headache, inflammation of the joints, etc. It will take more than 4 to 5 hours to get back to normal. Therefore, fasting 12 to 18 hours a day a week (or whenever you consume excessively) is a fantastic way to allow the body to return to its normal state to function naturally. This will create more energy by releasing the body from foods that interfere with its natural flow and cleanse or detoxify the liver and blood from unwanted nutrients.

So, if you have more energy for your desire, consider these recommendations in your daily diet. Take one or two or all the tips and have them work for you. I think you'll notice a difference in how you feel and how your body works. We must all return to the basics of life and remember what triggered the behaviour of our teenagers! You may need the motivation to help you.

➢ Lessons on Intermittent Years of Fasting:

1. Sometimes fasting is not a "starvation" diet; It's a healthy lifestyle.

Whenever an average person first learns about the occasional fast, he/she usually says, "Oh yes, I already did it, you mean hungry for weight loss, right?"

Sometimes fasting is a way of life. It's a lifestyle you could maintain throughout your life.

The by-product is weight loss, improvement of mental and physical health, etc. So far, the occasional fast has not been detrimental to my health. My health has improved considerably over time.

2. Listen to Your Body to Find Out What You Should Eat:

One of the most common questions about fasting is the occasional fasting diet. But as I already explained, it's not a diet, in fact it's a diet and lifestyle model.

During the feeding window, you can eat any combination of healthy foods.

The most important lesson I learned about "what to eat" is to listen to your body and eat accordingly.

For example, if you feel tired and exhausted after eating rice or cereal, you can try eating more vegetables. If you feel more energetic, then your body advises you to stick to vegetables and avoid eating foods high in carbohydrates.

That's why I am strongly encouraged by a "fixed" regime. Our body constantly changes as we get older, and eating the same foods every day increases the risk of developing food intolerance and disease.

Fortunately, I came across this idea of "eating while listening to your body" by reading the work of Paul Chek, a world-renowned expert in the field of health, in my book Eating, Moving, and Being Healthy.

The key lesson here is to continually listen to your body and experiment with different foods for optimal health.

3. The Advantage of Occasional Fasting: Simplify Your Life:

Before intermittent fasting, I was obsessed with getting up early to prepare breakfast, preparing six meals a day, and so on.

Although I have made some progress in achieving my health goals (fat loss, muscle gain, etc.), I struggled to stay consistent because this routine was tedious.

Today, life is much simpler for me. I eat one or two main meals a day, I'm not obsessed with what I eat, and I continue to progress each day to improve my strength and health.

Simplifying my life in this way has freed more time and energy to focus on what is important to me.

4. Expect Your Results to Decrease After a Year or More:

During the first year of casual fasting, in 2013, I lost a lot of fat and put myself in the best shape of my life.

But after my first year, weight and fat loss was significantly reduced until I noticed no significant differences.

This makes sense because your body can lose only too much fat without harming your health.

5. Intermittent Fasting and High-Intensity Internet Training Equate to Rapid Fat Loss:

If you want to lose weight as quickly as possible, I recommend you introduce any form of high-intensity workout. For example, when I started with the occasional fast, I introduced 10 minutes of running three times a week, plus weekly football games.

You can select what you like to do, for example. Swim, jump, run and then increase the intensity until you run out of fuel after each workout.

Also, training on an empty stomach also helped me improve my results. I'm not sure of the science that explains why fasting leads to fat loss, but I recommend you to experience it.

Intuitively, it makes sense to know why it works. Fasting helps reduce the number of calories you consume, while high-intensity workouts burn more calories. Your daily caloric intake drops significantly, and you lose more fat over time. Simple!

6. Sometimes Fasting Can Improve Your Discipline, Concentration, and Productivity:

During the fast, until 1 pm, I work much more than if I had lunch when I woke up. Once I break down quickly with my first meal, my energy level goes down, I lose focus and feel lethargic.

For this reason, I plan my most important tasks before arriving at my publication. This allows me to align my highest energy levels to my top most priorities, which translate into high productivity.

Another conclusion I have noticed is that the discipline of fasting has dramatically improved my training daily for the rest of my life. Once I started an informal publication, I developed a desire to make new habits: eat healthily, sleep early, read more, etc.

This is the power of the keystone habit.

7. Sometimes Fasting Can Reduce Your Discipline, Concentration and Productivity:

This may seem different to the previous point, but think about it, a hungry man can also be a hateful man. In other words, when you fast, it's easy to lose concentration and get angry because you're starving. That's why it's so essential to listen to your body and not stick to a fixed diet.

I noticed that there is an ideal area every day, a period to stop the publication window.

If you stop smoking too quickly, you will run out of energy that could be used to do more work.

If it breaks, you will get angry too late, and you will lose your concentration throughout the day.

Every day is different, so it's a trial and a mistake.

8. Intermittent Fasting Can Make Your Diet Worse:

After the previous point, when you are dying of hunger and you explode quickly, it is easy to eat unhealthy or nutritious empty foods. It was one of my biggest challenges with the occasional release.

Human discipline must fast daily. But superhuman control is necessary to obtain and maintain a healthy diet every day. The reason is that when you fast, your body weakens with sugar and energy. It is also hungry for foods rich in carbohydrates containing sugar. Although you can still achieve your weight and aesthetic goals without a healthy diet, in the long run, this can be harmful to your health.

The best way I've found to avoid this tendency to overeat after a rapid decline is to design my environment to succeed and drink as much water as possible throughout the day.

9. Intermittent Fasting Can Contribute to Losing or Gaining Muscle Mass:

Throughout my second year of intermittent fasting, I wounded my lower back with squats on my back and told myself not to lift weights indefinitely. I was already in shape, and I understood that everything would remain the same. So I substituted my weight training with Pilates and stretching exercises. I also started a body detox program, which included eliminating high carbohydrate foods from my diet for several months.

In a few weeks, my muscle mass had decreased so much that my clothes did not fit me anymore. The detox program and the intermittent fasting protocol had significantly reduced my daily calorie intake, contributing to muscle loss. After recovering, I resumed my bodybuilding program and increased my carbohydrate intake while maintaining the intermittent fasting protocol. In a few months, I regained my fitness and developed the muscles that I had initially lost.

The main lesson is that calorie intake is essential, a lot!

10. Intermittent Fasting Works Because You Take Fewer Calories:

Like any novice, during the first year of casual fasting, I thought I had discovered the magic formula for losing weight and leading a healthy life. I would tell everyone that this was the only way to achieve their health goals because it worked very well for me.

Over the years, as I have experienced more often, I have discovered that the reason intermittent fasting can be so beneficial for weight loss is simply that it requires less food. The less you eat, the fewer calories you consume and the more pounds you lose.

It's that simple. It's not magic.

Some people who try to end the fast reject it by complaining that it does not work. But in most cases, they could not track their caloric intake. Intermittent fasting is just another tool to help you reduce your caloric intake. But if you decide to eat junk food after each message, you can put on weight as before. In other words, as I said before, the amount of calories you consume each day is significant.

Continuous fasting should not be used as an excuse to savour your favourite ice cream or lose discipline while eating well. For this reason, you can achieve your health goals by eating six or more meals a day. As long as the total number of calories you consume each day is less than what you use to move and live, you will lose weight over time.

11. Do not Let the Occasional Fast Stop You from Living Your Life:

The biggest lesson I learned during my four-year hike is not to worry about what's perfect and live your life alone. During my first year, I refused to go quickly through the window to eat. I was travelling on vacation to new places, avoiding the experience of trying fresh foods from a different culture because of fasting.

I used to be severe and categorical about my occasional fasting protocol. But over time, I've learned that life is not just about achieving your goals of training, nutrition, or fitness. I'm still working to reach my health goals every week, but I'm not penalized if I'm not responsible.

Sometimes, I eat breakfast instead of fasting while sometimes, I stop fasting at the right time but eat unhealthy foods.

www.ingramcontent.com/pod-product-compliance
Lightning Source LLC
Chambersburg PA
CBHW070830250726
48662CB00003B/1151